Chair Yoga

For Seniors

A Gentle Guide To Flexibility, Balance, Renewed
Strength And Vitality

Nardine Brown

ISBN: 9798325544804

DEDICATION

To Katherine, for your love and faithfulness.

TABLE OF CONTENTS

CHAPTER 1: INTRODUCTION

Welcome to the wonderful world of chair yoga! This gentle practice is designed specifically for seniors, offering a safe and effective way to improve your flexibility, strength, balance and overall well-being. Whether you're new to yoga or have experience on the mat, chair yoga provides a unique opportunity to enjoy the benefits of yoga while remaining comfortably seated or supported by a chair.

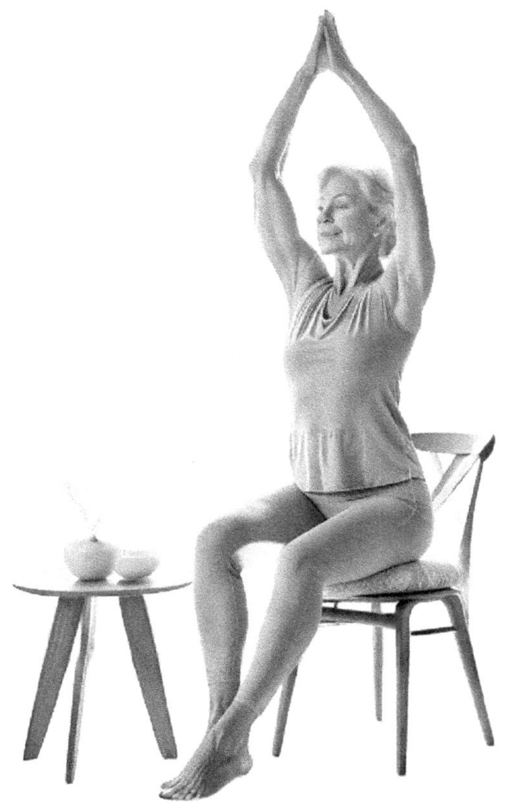

This book will be your guide to exploring the many ways chair yoga can enrich your life. We'll explore the fundamentals of chair yoga postures, breathing techniques and the positive impact this practice can have on your physical and mental health. As you embark on this journey, you'll discover a newfound sense of ease in movement, improved coordination and a boost in your mood.

Throughout this book, we'll provide clear instructions for each pose, along with modifications to ensure you can tailor the practice to your specific needs and abilities. Remember, there's no competition in chair yoga. It's all about listening to your body and enjoying the process of mindful movement.

So, get ready to embrace a more vibrant and fulfilling life! With chair yoga as your companion, you'll be well on your way to achieving greater strength, flexibility, and a renewed sense of inner peace.

What is Chair Yoga?

Chair yoga is a welcoming and adaptable form of yoga designed specifically for those who prefer to practice while seated or with the help of a chair for balance. It allows you to experience the many benefits of yoga, regardless of your physical limitations or experience level.

Imagine a yoga practice tailored to your comfort, where poses are modified or done entirely while seated. Chair yoga provides a safe and supported environment to improve your flexibility, strength, and overall well-being.

Here are some key aspects of chair yoga:

- **Focus on seated postures:** Most poses are done while seated in a sturdy chair with good back support.
- **Chair for balance:** The chair is used as an extension of your body, offering support and stability for standing poses or stretches.
- **Gentle movements:** Chair yoga emphasizes gentle movements that are easy on your joints.
- **Breathing exercises:** Just like traditional yoga, chair yoga incorporates mindful breathing techniques to promote relaxation and focus.

Whether you're a seasoned yogi or just starting your fitness journey, chair yoga gives you a gentle and effective way to enhance your physical and mental well-being. This book will guide you through a variety of chair yoga poses specifically designed for seniors, helping you find renewed strength, flexibility and a sense of calm.

Who Is Chair Yoga For?

Chair yoga is for everyone! It's a gentle and adaptable practice that offers a wealth of benefits, especially for seniors. Whether you're a seasoned yogi or just starting your fitness journey, chair yoga provides a safe and supportive environment to improve your overall well-being.

Chair yoga is particularly beneficial for seniors who:

- Have limited mobility or difficulty getting down on the floor.
- Are recovering from surgery or an injury.
- Manage chronic health conditions.
- Want to improve their balance and coordination.
- Seek a gentle form of exercise to promote overall well-being.

No matter your age or fitness level, chair yoga provides a welcoming and effective way to move your body, improve your health, and find inner peace.

Chair yoga is a gentle and adaptable practice for seniors, even those managing specific health conditions or recovering from injuries. This chapter will explore how chair yoga can be tailored to address some common concerns. Remember, it's crucial to listen to your body and consult with your doctor before starting any new exercise program, especially if you have any pre-existing conditions.

Arthritis and Joint Pain:

- **Focus:** Gentle movements to improve flexibility and reduce stiffness.
- **Modifications:** Avoid poses that put stress on weight-bearing joints. Opt for seated arm circles, chair stretches, and seated toe raises instead.
- **Benefits:** Improved range of motion, reduced pain and increased joint lubrication.

Balance Issues:

- **Focus:** Poses that challenge proprioception (body awareness) and improve balance.
- **Modifications:** Begin with poses with hand support on the chair for stability. Gradually progress to standing poses with light chair support. Practice heel-toe walking while seated.
- **Benefits:** Enhanced balance and reduced risk of falls.

Cardiovascular Health:

- **Focus:** Low-impact movements that elevate heart rate moderately.
- **Modifications:** Seated arm raises, leg extensions, and torso twists can be incorporated with rhythmic breathing.
- **Benefits:** Improved circulation, heart health, and overall well-being.

Lower Back Pain:

- **Focus:** Strengthening core muscles and improving spinal alignment.
- **Modifications:** Avoid poses that twist or strain the lower back. Focus on seated cat-cow stretches, pelvic tilts, and seated glute squeezes.
- **Benefits:** Reduced pain, improved core strength, and better posture.

Osteoporosis:

- **Focus:** Weight-bearing exercises to improve bone density.
- **Modifications:** Seated leg press against a resistance band, seated calf raises, and chair squats with support are excellent options.
- **Benefits:** Increased bone strength and reduced risk of fractures.

Remember:

- **Listen to your body:** Pain is a signal to stop or modify the pose.
- **Start slow and gradually increase intensity:** Don't push yourself beyond your limits.
- **Focus on proper form:** Alignment is key to preventing injuries.
- **Enjoy the practice:** Chair yoga is a journey, not a destination. Focus on the mindful movements and the joy of movement.

Additional Tips:

- Utilize props like yoga blocks, straps, and cushions for added support and comfort.
- Breathe deeply with a steady rhythm throughout each pose.
- Practice regularly for optimal benefits.

Disclaimer: This information is for educational purposes only and should not be a substitute for professional medical advice. Always consult with your doctor before starting a new exercise program.

The Benefits Of Chair Yoga For Seniors

As we age, staying active and keeping our bodies limber becomes even more important. Chair yoga gives seniors a fantastic way to reap the benefits of yoga, without the need for getting down on the floor or strenuous poses.

Here's how chair yoga can be a game-changer for seniors:

Enhanced Flexibility and Range of Motion: Sitting for long periods can tighten muscles and limit movement. Chair yoga incorporates gentle stretches that target different muscle groups, helping seniors reach further, twist easier and bend with more confidence. This improved flexibility makes daily activities like dressing, gardening or even reaching for groceries on high shelves much simpler.

Building Strength for Better Balance: Chair yoga may seem gentle, but don't underestimate its power to build strength. Many poses use the chair for support while engaging core muscles and major muscle groups in the arms and legs. This newfound strength translates into better balance, which can significantly reduce the risk of falls, a common concern for seniors.

Improved Coordination and Body Awareness: Chair yoga poses often involve reaching, twisting, and controlled movements while seated or using the chair for stability. This focus on coordination helps seniors become more aware of their body's position in space, leading to smoother transitions during daily activities and a reduced risk of bumps or awkward movements.

Stress Reduction and Mental Well-being: Yoga is well-known for its ability to promote relaxation and mindfulness. Chair yoga is no different. The practice of focusing on breath and gentle movements helps quiet the mind, reduce stress and anxiety, and elevate mood. This mental well-being can contribute to better sleep quality and an overall sense of calmness.

Reduced Pain and Improved Pain Management: For seniors dealing with arthritis or chronic pain, chair yoga is a low-impact way to move their bodies without aggravating discomfort. The gentle stretches can help improve blood flow to stiff joints, reduce pain intensity, and even increase pain tolerance.

Social Connection and Fun: Chair yoga classes can be a great way for seniors to socialize and connect with others in a supportive environment. The camaraderie and shared experience can boost mood, combat feelings of isolation, and make exercise more enjoyable.

Getting Started With Chair Yoga

The beauty of chair yoga is that it's accessible to almost everyone, regardless of fitness level or physical limitations. A sturdy chair is all you need to get started. Here are some tips:

- **Consult with your doctor:** Before beginning any new exercise program, especially if you have any health concerns, it's important to get your doctor's approval.
- **Find a qualified instructor:** Look for classes specifically designed for chair yoga or seniors. A certified instructor can modify poses for individual needs and ensure proper form to avoid injury.
- **Listen to your body:** Don't push yourself beyond your limits. Chair yoga should be gentle and enjoyable.

- **Focus on your breath:** Breathe deeply and slowly throughout each pose to maximize relaxation and mindfulness.

Chair yoga is a wonderful way for seniors to stay active, improve their overall well-being, and embrace a healthy and fulfilling lifestyle.

CHAPTER 2: GETTING READY

Approaching Chair Yoga with the Perfect Mindset

Chair yoga is a fantastic practice for people of all ages and abilities. But before you dive into those stretches, setting the right intention in your mind can make all the difference. Here's how to cultivate a positive mindset for a truly enriching chair yoga experience:

1. Let Go of Expectations: This isn't a competition! Chair yoga is about connecting with your body in the present moment. Ditch any preconceived notions of how flexible you "should" be, and focus on gentle exploration instead.

2. Embrace Curiosity: Approach chair yoga with an open mind. There might be poses that feel unfamiliar or challenging at first. Instead of getting discouraged, view them as opportunities to learn about your body's unique capabilities.

3. Celebrate Small Victories: Even the tiniest improvements are worth acknowledging. Did your balance feel a little steadier today? Did you reach a bit further in a side bend? Take a moment to appreciate your progress, no matter how small.

4. Kindness is Key: Be gentle with yourself throughout the practice. There will be days when certain poses feel more difficult. Instead of pushing yourself to the point of discomfort, listen to your body and adjust accordingly. Remember, yoga is about self-care, not self-punishment.

5. Find Your Breath: Yoga and breath are like two peas in a pod. Focus on your breath during each pose. As you inhale, imagine drawing in fresh energy. As you exhale, let go of any tension or worries. By synchronizing your breath with movement, you'll find a deeper sense of calm and focus.

6. Embrace Gratitude: Take a moment at the beginning or end of your practice to express gratitude for your body. Thank it for carrying you through life's journey. This simple act can foster a deeper appreciation for your physical wellbeing.

7. Make it Yours: Don't be afraid to personalize your chair yoga experience. If a particular pose feels uncomfortable, modify it! Find what works best for you and your body. You can even add some soothing music or light some calming aromatherapy candles to create a truly restorative environment.

8. Be Present: Chair yoga is a wonderful opportunity to practice mindfulness. Focus on the sensations in your body as you move. Notice the rise and fall of your chest with each breath. By quieting your mind and tuning into the present moment, you'll unlock a world of relaxation and inner peace.

Remember: The most important aspect of chair yoga is to find joy in the practice. Let go of any pressure to perform perfectly, and simply enjoy the gentle movements and mindful breathing. By approaching chair yoga with the right mindset, you'll transform it from a simple exercise routine into a journey of self-discovery and well-being.

Chair yoga is a wonderful way to experience the benefits of yoga poses without needing to get down on the floor. It's a great option for beginners, people with limitations, or anyone who wants a gentler yoga practice. Here's what you'll need to get started:

Equipment:

- **Sturdy chair:** This is the most important piece of equipment for chair yoga. Look for a chair with a firm seat and back and good back support. Ideally, the chair should be armless so you can move your arms freely during poses. However, a chair with arms can be helpful for providing extra stability in some balancing postures.
- **Yoga mat (optional):** While not essential, a yoga mat can provide extra cushioning and grip on the floor if you need to step down for certain poses that involve reaching the floor slightly. It can also help define your practice area and add a touch of comfort, especially if your floor is on the cold side.
- **Comfortable clothing:** Wear loose-fitting clothing that allows for easy movement. Opt for natural fabrics like cotton or linen that will breathe well as you move your body.

Space Setup:

- **Find a quiet and clear space:** Look for a spot in your home where you can move freely without bumping into furniture or walls. There should be enough room to comfortably extend your arms and legs out to the sides and forward.
- **Clear away tripping hazards:** Make sure the floor is free of clutter, rugs, or anything else that you could trip over during your practice.

- **Lighting and ventilation:** Choose a well-lit and ventilated area. You want to be able to see yourself clearly and adjust your posture if needed. Good ventilation will help keep you cool and comfortable, especially if you tend to get warm during exercise.
- **Wall for support (optional):** Having a wall nearby can be helpful for providing extra support during balancing poses. If you decide you want the option of using a wall for support, position your chair a few feet away from it.
- **Chair height adjustment:** Before you begin your practice, adjust the chair height so that your feet rest flat on the floor with your knees bent at a 90-degree angle when you sit down. This will help ensure proper posture and alignment throughout your practice.

Additional Tips:

- You can add some extra props to your chair yoga routine to enhance your practice or modify poses for your needs. A yoga strap can help you improve your flexibility in certain poses, while light weights can add a little extra challenge for strength building.
- If you're new to chair yoga, it's a good idea to find a chair yoga class or video led by a certified instructor. This will help you learn proper form and technique to get the most out of your practice.

With a little bit of preparation, you can easily create a safe and comfortable space for your chair yoga practice at home.

Chair yoga is a fantastic way to experience the benefits of yoga, regardless of age, fitness level, or physical limitations. But like any exercise, it's important to prioritize safety to get the most out of your practice and avoid injuries. Here are some key tips and precautions to keep in mind:

Before You Begin:

- **Listen to your body:** If you have any pre-existing injuries or medical conditions, consult your doctor before starting chair yoga. Discuss any limitations you might have and get their guidance on modifications for specific poses.
- **Choose the right chair:** Look for a sturdy chair with a flat, stable base and a backrest that offers some support but allows for upright posture. Avoid chairs with wheels, swivel mechanisms, or armrests that could get in the way. A chair with a slightly firm seat cushion is ideal for providing good balance.

Setting Up Your Practice Space:

- **Find a clear area:** Make sure you have enough space around your chair to move comfortably without bumping into furniture or walls. Ideally, practice on a non-slip surface like a yoga mat or carpeted area to prevent falls.

Safety During Practice:

- **Focus on proper form:** Don't push yourself beyond your limits. Chair yoga is about gentle movements and stretches, not about achieving perfect poses. Pay attention to your instructor's cues and prioritize proper body alignment to avoid strain or discomfort.

- **Maintain good posture:** Sit tall with your shoulders relaxed and back straight. Keep your core engaged and feet placed flat on the floor, hip-width apart. This will provide a stable base for your movements.
- **Move slowly and mindfully:** Avoid jerky or bouncing motions. Focus on smooth, controlled movements while coordinating your breath with each pose. Inhale as you open your body and exhale as you release or fold.
- **Listen to your body:** Pain is a signal to stop. If you feel any pain or discomfort during a pose, gently come out of it and rest. There are always modifications you can make to accommodate your individual needs.
- **Don't hold your breath:** Breathe deeply and evenly throughout your practice. Holding your breath can restrict oxygen flow and lead to dizziness.
- **Stay hydrated:** Drink plenty of water before, during, and after your chair yoga session, especially in hot or humid environments.
- **Be aware of your surroundings:** If you're practicing in a group class, be mindful of other students and their space.

Additional Precautions:

- **Balance:** If you have concerns about balance, consider placing a hand on the chair seat for additional support during standing poses.
- **High blood pressure:** Inversions (poses where the head is below the heart) and deep twists are not recommended for people with high blood pressure. Opt for gentle stretches and seated twists instead.
- **Dizziness:** If you start to feel lightheaded or dizzy during any pose, come out of it slowly and sit down until the feeling passes.

Remember: Chair yoga is a journey, not a destination. It's about enjoying the gentle movements, improving flexibility, and finding inner peace. By following these safety tips and precautions, you can create a safe and enjoyable chair yoga practice that benefits your body and mind.

Talking to Your Doctor Before You Start Chair Yoga

Chair yoga is a fantastic way to improve your flexibility, balance, and overall well-being. But even though it's gentle and uses a chair for support, it's always a good idea to chat with your doctor before you dive into a new exercise routine. Here's why:

Safety First:

- **Pre-existing Conditions:** Some health issues, like heart problems, arthritis, or balance issues, might need modifications or a different type of exercise altogether. Your doctor can give you the green light and recommend any adjustments needed to keep you safe and comfortable.
- **Medications:** Certain medications can affect your balance or blood pressure. Your doctor can advise you on how chair yoga might interact with your medications and if there's anything to watch out for.
- **Recent Injuries:** If you've had a recent surgery or injury, your doctor can help you determine if chair yoga is appropriate and suggest any limitations to avoid further problems.

Getting the Most Out of Chair Yoga

- **Tailored Recommendations:** Your doctor might know about specific chair yoga classes or resources that cater to people with similar health conditions to yours. This can help you find a program that's a perfect fit for your needs.
- **Modifications:** Some yoga poses might need tweaking depending on your abilities. Your doctor can help you understand which modifications are best for you to ensure you're getting the most benefit and avoiding any discomfort.

- **Gradual Progression:** Even chair yoga can be a bit challenging initially. Your doctor can advise you on a safe starting point and a gradual progression plan to help you build your strength and flexibility without overdoing it.

What to Discuss with Your Doctor:

- Briefly explain what chair yoga is and why you're interested in starting it.
- Mention any pre-existing health conditions, surgeries, or injuries you have.
- List any medications you're currently taking.
- Ask about any specific recommendations or modifications you might need.

Remember, your doctor is your partner in health. By having a quick conversation beforehand, you can ensure chair yoga becomes a safe and enjoyable way to improve your well-being.

CHAPTER 3: BREATHING AND WARM-UP

Warming Up for Chair Yoga

Just like any other form of exercise, a proper warm-up is crucial before diving into your chair yoga routine. It prepares your body for movement, increases blood flow, and helps prevent injuries. Here's how to get your body ready for a safe and enjoyable chair yoga session:

Settle In and Find Your Breath (5 minutes)

1. **Sit comfortably:** Choose a sturdy chair with good back support. Sit tall with both feet placed flat on the floor, hip-width apart.
2. **Center yourself:** Breathe deeply a few times in through your nose and exhale slowly out through your mouth. Feel your belly rise and fall with each breath. Focus on calming your mind and releasing any tension.

Gentle Neck and Spine Mobilizations (5 minutes)

1. **Neck rolls:** Slowly roll your head in a circular motion, tracing large circles with your chin first one way, then the other. Do 5-10 rolls in each direction.
2. **Lateral neck stretches:** Gently tilt your ear towards your shoulder, feeling a stretch along the side of your neck. Hold for 10-15 seconds, then repeat the stretch on the other side.
3. **Spinal twists:** Sit with your feet placed flat on the floor. Inhale and lengthen your spine. Exhale and twist your torso gently to one side, looking over your shoulder. Hold for 10-15 seconds, then repeat the twist on the other side.

Waking Up Your Upper Body (5 minutes)

1. **Arm circles:** Sit tall and extend your arms straight out to the sides at shoulder height. Make small circles forward for 10 repetitions, and then reverse directions for another 10.
2. **Shoulder rolls:** Lift your shoulders and roll them forward in a circular motion 5 times, then reverse directions and roll them backward 5 times.
3. **Eagle arms:** Cross your forearms at the front of your chest, elbows bent at 90 degrees. Wrap your forearms around each other, bringing your palms together (or as close as comfortable). Gently lift your arms overhead and hold for 10-15 seconds. Reverse the position of your arms and repeat.

Warming Up Your Lower Body (5 minutes)

1. **Ankle circles:** Sit tall and lift one foot off the floor. Rotate your ankle in circles 5 times in each direction. Repeat with the other foot.
2. **Calf raises:** Sit with both feet placed flat on the floor. Lift your heels off the ground, raising yourself onto the balls of your feet. Hold for a few seconds, then lower your heels back down. Repeat 10-15 times.
3. **Knee circles:** Sit tall and extend one leg out straight in front of you. Make small circles with your foot, clockwise for 5 repetitions, then counter-clockwise for 5 repetitions. Repeat with the other leg.

Remember:

- Listen to your body. Move slowly and with intention throughout the warm-up.
- Breathe deeply and continuously throughout all the exercises.
- Don't push yourself into any position that causes pain.
- Modify any exercises as needed to suit your limitations.

This is just a sample warm-up routine. Feel free to adjust it based on your needs and preferences. You can also find many guided chair yoga warm-up videos online [YouTube] for a more visual demonstration.

By taking the time to warm up properly, you'll be setting yourself up for a successful and enjoyable chair yoga practice!

Breathing Exercises For Chair Yoga

Chair yoga provides a fantastic way to improve flexibility, balance, and strength from the comfort of a chair. But did you know that focusing on your breath can elevate your chair yoga practice even further? Breathing exercises, also known as pranayama in yoga, make you more aware of your breath, improve oxygen flow, and enhance the connection between mind and body. Here are some powerful breathing techniques you can integrate into your chair yoga routine:

1. Slow and Steady: Dirga Swasham (Three-Part Breath)

1. Sit comfortably with a tall spine and feet placed flat on the floor (or on yoga blocks for added height).
2. Place one hand on your belly and the other on your chest.
3. Inhale through your nose slowly, feeling your belly expand first (like a balloon inflating) followed by your chest rising gently.
4. Exhale through pursed lips slowly, feeling your belly deflate first and then your chest sinking down.
5. Count silently to a comfortable number for your inhale (perhaps 4 seconds) and another comfortable number for your exhale (maybe 6 seconds).
6. Repeat this breath for several cycles, focusing on the smooth, rhythmic movement of your belly and chest.

2. Energizing Breath: Kapalbhati (Bellows Breath)

1. Sit with a tall spine and take a quick, forceful exhale through your nose, contracting your abdominal muscles as you push the air out.
2. Inhale passively, letting your belly fill naturally.
3. Repeat this sequence of forceful exhales and passive inhales in a rapid, rhythmic way for a short period (around 10-15 breaths).
4. Breathe normally for a few breaths afterward to rebalance your energy.

3. Calming Breath: Bhramari Pranayama (Bee Breath)

1. Sit comfortably and close your eyes or soften your gaze.
2. Pinch your nostrils shut with your thumb and index finger.
3. Inhale through your nose deeply (even though your nostrils are closed, you should still feel a slight sensation of air entering).
4. As you exhale, make a gentle humming sound like a bee.
5. Repeat this cycle of inhaling through the nose (with nostrils closed) and exhaling with a bee hum for several breaths.

4. Cooling Breath: Sitali Pranayama (Cooling Breath)

1. Sit comfortably and close your eyes or soften your gaze.
2. Curl your tongue into a U-shape, like a taco.
3. Inhale deeply through your curled tongue, feeling the cool air fill your lungs.
4. Close your mouth then exhale slowly through your nose.
5. Repeat this cycle of inhaling through your curled tongue and exhaling through your nose for several breaths.

Remember:

- Pay attention to your body and adjust the breathing exercises to feel comfortable.
- If you sense any dizziness, slow down or stop the exercise.

- Coordinate your breath with your chair yoga movements. For example, inhale as you reach your arms overhead and exhale as you fold forward.

By incorporating these breathing exercises into your chair yoga routine, you'll not only improve your physical well-being but also cultivate a sense of focus and calmness within.

CHAPTER 4: BEGINNER CHAIR YOGA POSES

Stepping into the world of yoga can feel intimidating, but chair yoga tones down this intimidation by offering a gentle and accessible way to experience its benefits. Even if your mobility is limited or you are new to exercise, chair yoga allows you to practice yoga poses from the comfort and support of a chair. This beginner-friendly routine focuses on basic movements that improve flexibility, strengthen core muscles, and enhance balance. All you need is a sturdy chair and a willingness to explore! Let's begin your chair yoga journey with some fundamental poses that will leave you feeling refreshed and invigorated.

Chair Mountain Pose (Tadasana)

The Chair Mountain Pose, also known as Tadasana in Sanskrit, is the foundation of many chair yoga poses. It promotes proper posture and body awareness, thereby setting the stage for your practice. Here's how to find stability and stillness in this pose:

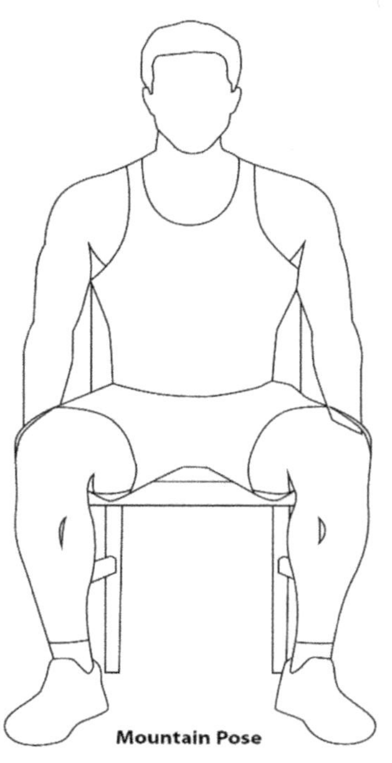

1. Begin by sitting on a sturdy chair with feet placed flat on the floor, at about hip-width apart. Avoid slouching – lengthen your spine by imagining your head being gently pulled upwards.
2. Gently draw your belly button inwards, engaging your core

muscles. This provides stability and helps maintain proper alignment throughout your body.

3. Press your feet into the floor firmly, feeling all your toes grounded. Imagine pushing the floor away with your soles to activate your leg muscles.
4. Gently open your chest by rolling your shoulders back and down. Avoid hunching your shoulders forward. Maintain a relaxed yet lifted posture in your upper body.
5. Soften your gaze by looking slightly forward or upwards. Avoid straining your neck by keeping your head in a natural, comfortable position.
6. Inhale through the nose, slowly and deeply feeling your belly expand. Exhale slowly through the mouth, releasing any tension. Focus on your breath and how it connects to your movements.

Hold Chair Mountain Pose for several breaths, allowing your body to settle into a comfortable and stable position. This pose is a great starting point for your chair yoga practice, and you can revisit it throughout your routine to check in with your alignment and breath.

Chair Cat-Cow Pose (Marjaryasana-Bitilasana)

The Chair Cat-Cow Pose, a combination of Marjaryasana (Cat Pose) and Bitilasana (Cow Pose), gently stretches and mobilizes your spine. It improves flexibility and encourages healthy blood flow. Here's how to move gracefully through this pose:

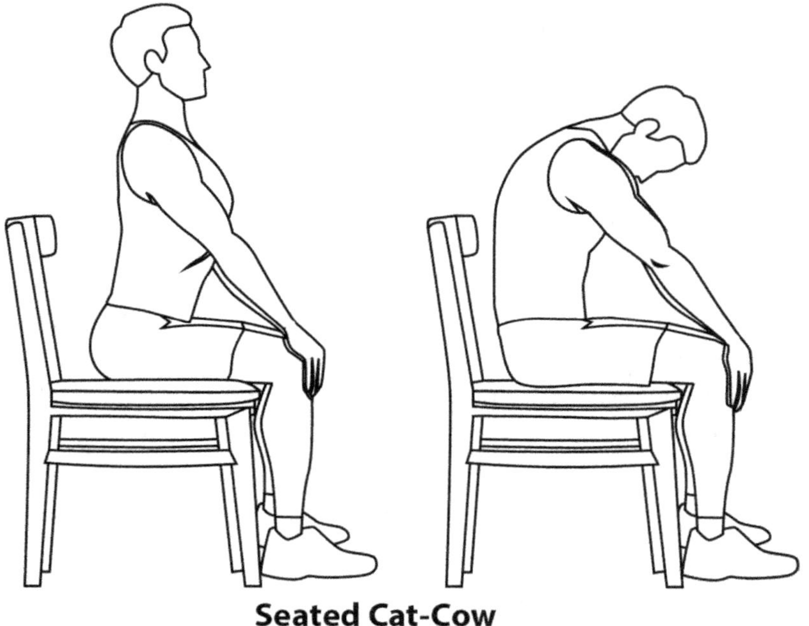

Seated Cat-Cow

1. Sit comfortably on your chair with feet placed flat on the floor, at about hip-width apart. Place your hands lightly on your thighs or knees.
2. As you inhale, gently arch your back, then lift your chest and head slightly upwards. Engage your core muscles to maintain a neutral lower back. Imagine your belly button drawing inwards towards your spine.
3. As you are exhaling, round your spine, and tuck your chin in towards your chest. Let your shoulder blades gently come together and feel a gentle stretch in your lower back.
4. Continue inhaling for the cow pose and then exhaling for the cat pose, finding a smooth, rhythmic movement in your

breath and spine. Repeat this cycle for several breaths, focusing on the gentle stretch and release in your back.

Chair Forward Bend/Fold (Uttanasana)

The Chair Forward Bend, also known as Uttanasana, stretches your hamstrings, back, and shoulders, promoting flexibility and relaxation. Here's how to find a comfortable forward bend with the support of your chair:

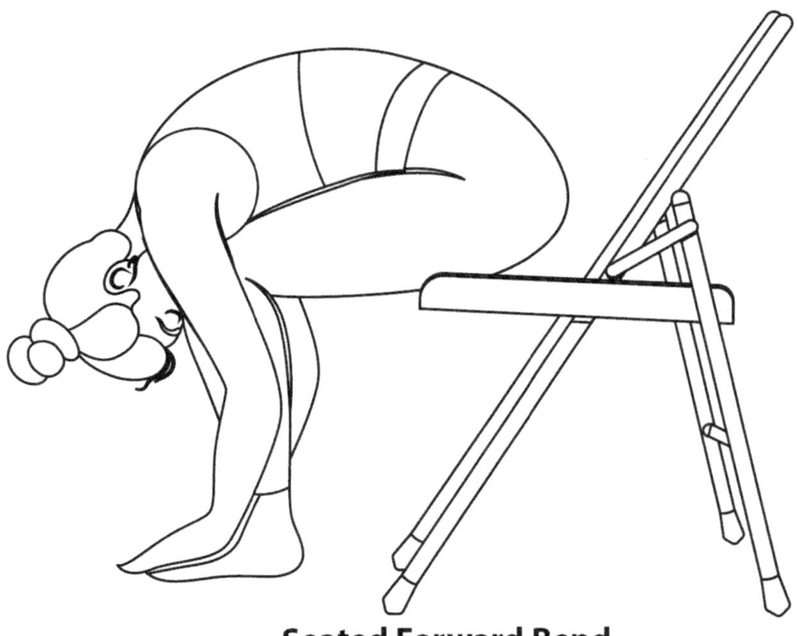

Seated Forward Bend

1. Sit tall on your chair with feet placed flat on the floor, at about hip-width apart. Engage your core muscles then lengthen your spine by reaching the crown of your head upwards.
2. Take a deep inhale and reach your arms overhead, lengthening your spine further. Palms can face each other or be turned upwards.

3. As you exhale, hinge at the hips and gently fold forward, reaching your hands towards the floor. If comfortable, rest your hands on the floor or your shins. Keep your back long and avoid rounding your shoulders.

4. Concentrate on lengthening your spine rather than forcing yourself to reach a certain point. You can adjust the position of your hands by placing them on the chair seat or behind your thighs if reaching the floor is difficult.

5. If comfortable, gently walk your fingertips down your shins or towards the floor as you exhale further. Keep your knees at a slight bend to avoid locking them.

6. Hold the forward bend for several breaths, focusing on your deep, rhythmic breathing. Feel the gentle stretch in your hamstrings, back, and shoulders.

7. To come out of this pose, inhale and slowly lengthen your spine back to the seated position. Bring down your arms alongside your body at your own pace.

Chair Arm Circles

Chair Arm Circles gently warm up your shoulders and improve upper body mobility. This is a great way to prepare your body for further movement in your chair yoga practice. Here's how to perform this energizing exercise:

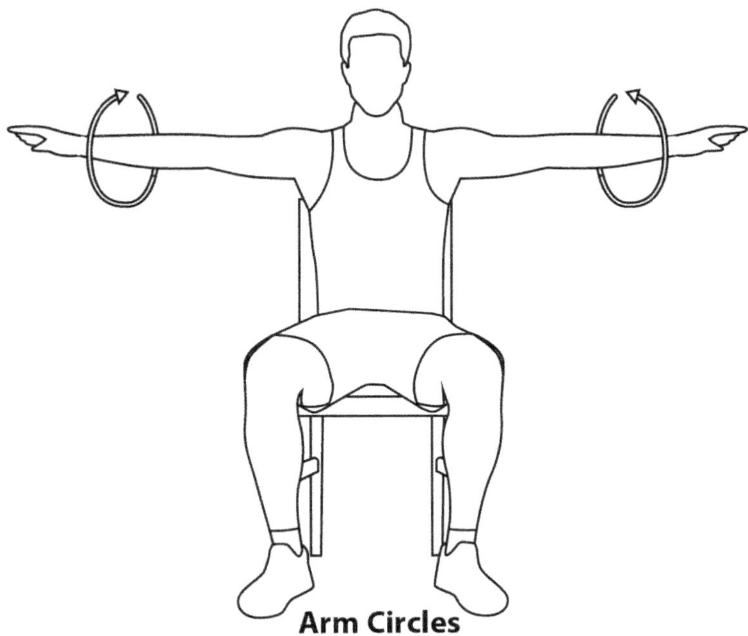

1. Sit comfortably on your chair with feet placed flat on the floor, at about hip-width apart. Maintain a tall spine and let your shoulders relax.
2. Extend your two arms out to the sides, keeping them straight or slightly bent at the elbows, palms facing down.
3. Begin making small circles with your arms, moving forward (toward your thumbs) for several breaths. Focus on relaxing your shoulders and engaging your midsection.
4. After completing your forward circles, switch directions and make small circles backward (toward your little fingers) for several breaths.

5. Continue alternating forward and backward circles for several cycles, finding a smooth rhythm in your movements. Breathe deeply throughout the exercise, feeling the gentle stretch in your shoulders and upper back.

Chair Neck Rolls

Neck rolls offer a simple yet effective way to release tension and improve mobility in your neck. Here's how to perform Chair Neck Rolls:

1. Begin by sitting comfortably on your chair with feet placed flat on the floor, at about hip-width apart. Maintain a tall spine with your shoulders relaxed.
2. Gently lower your chin towards your chest, starting the roll.
3. Begin rolling your head in a clockwise direction, making small circles. Let your head lead the movement, and avoid forcing it.
4. Continue the circle until your head returns to the starting position (facing forward with your chin tucked slightly).
5. Repeat the neck roll in a counter-clockwise direction, making small, controlled circles.
6. Perform a few sets of neck rolls in each direction (clockwise and counter-clockwise), breathing deeply throughout. Focus on the gentle stretch and release of any tension in your neck muscles.

Chair Yoga Neck Stretch

Gentle neck stretches can help alleviate tension and improve mobility in your neck and shoulders. Here are a few stretches you can perform while seated in your chair:

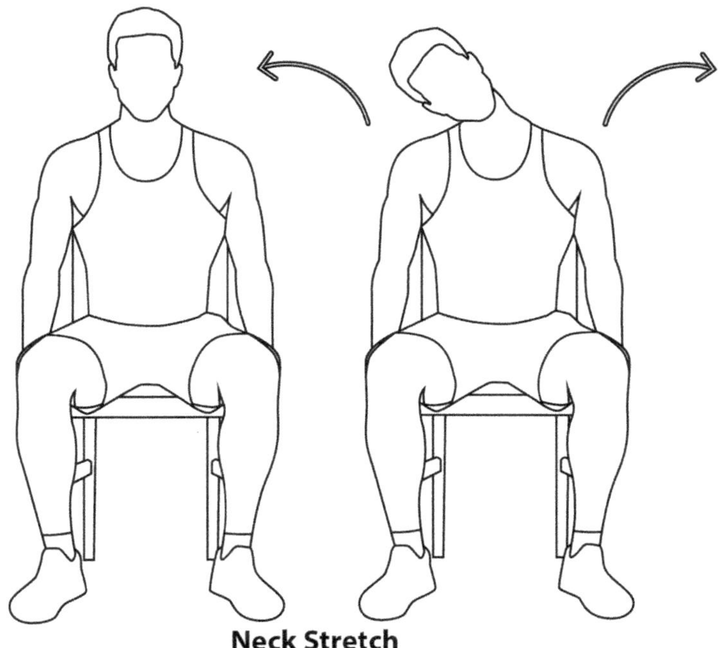

Neck Stretch

1. Sit comfortably on a chair with your feet flat on the ground and your spine tall.
2. Relax your shoulders down away from your ears, allowing your arms to rest comfortably by your sides.
3. Inhale deeply and as you exhale, slowly tilt your head towards the right, bringing your right ear towards your right shoulder. Avoid lifting the shoulder.
4. Hold this stretch for about 5 breaths, feeling a gentle stretch on your neck along the left side.
5. Inhale as you return your head to the center.
6. Exhale and repeat the stretch to the left side, bringing your left ear towards your left shoulder.

7. Hold the position for a few breaths, feeling the stretch all along the right side of the neck.
8. Inhale and return your head to the center.
9. Now, tilt your head forward, bringing your chin towards your chest, feeling the stretch along the back of the neck.
10. Hold the position for a few breaths, maintaining a gentle stretch.
11. Inhale and slowly lift your head back to the center.
12. Finally, tilt your head backward, gently lifting your chin towards the ceiling, feeling a stretch along the front of your neck.
13. Hold for a couple of breaths, being mindful not to strain your neck.
14. Inhale as you return your head to the center.

Chair Ankle Circles

Ankle circles are a simple yet effective means to warm up your ankles and improve their range of motion. This can benefit your overall balance and stability throughout your chair yoga practice. Here's how to perform Chair Ankle Circles:

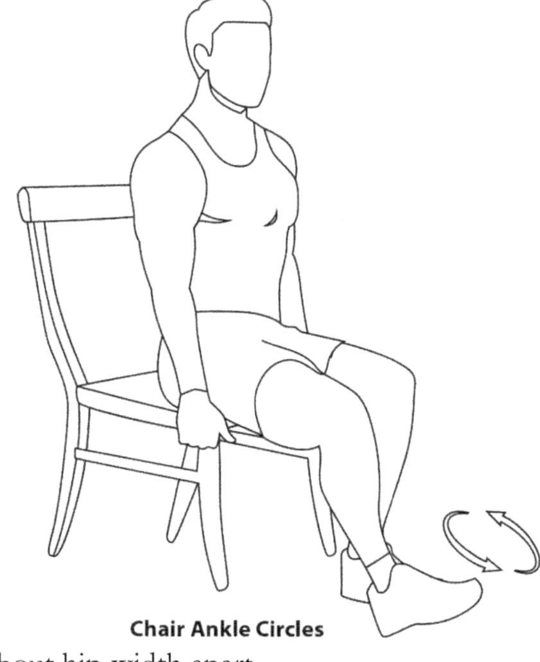

Chair Ankle Circles

1. Begin by sitting comfortably on your chair with feet placed flat on the floor, at about hip-width apart.
2. Start by pointing your toes out straight in front of you. Hold for a moment, then flex your feet, pulling your toes in towards your shins. Repeat this a few times to loosen up your ankle joints.
3. Now, keeping your toes pointed, slowly rotate your ankles in a clockwise direction. Make small circles for 5-10 repetitions.
4. Reverse direction and rotate your ankles in a counter-clockwise direction for another 5-10 repetitions.
5. Focus on the gentle movement in your ankles and any areas that feel tight. Breathe deeply throughout the circles.

Repeat steps 2-5 if you'd like to further warm up your ankles.

Chair Spinal Twist (Ardha Matsyendrasana)

The Chair Spinal Twist gently stretches and strengthens your core and back muscles while improving your range of motion in the spine. Here's how to find a comfortable twist in this pose:

Spinal Twist

1. Begin by sitting sideways on your chair with feet placed flat on the floor, at about hip-width apart.
2. Place your right hand behind you, palm flat, on the chair seat or the floor for added stability. Extend your left arm overhead, reaching towards the ceiling lengthen your spine.
3. Gently twist your torso towards the right, looking over your right shoulder. Engage your core muscles to maintain a stable and upright posture in your lower back.
4. Breathe deeply and comfortably while holding this twist for a few breaths. Feel the stretch along the spine and side waist.
5. Inhale as you slowly untwist your torso back to center. Repeat the twist on the other side, extending your left arm overhead and placing your right hand behind you for support. Breathe deeply and hold for a couple of breaths before slowly releasing.

Chair Side Stretch

The Chair Side Stretch helps improve flexibility in your side body and encourages good posture. Here's how to find a gentle side stretch while seated in your chair:

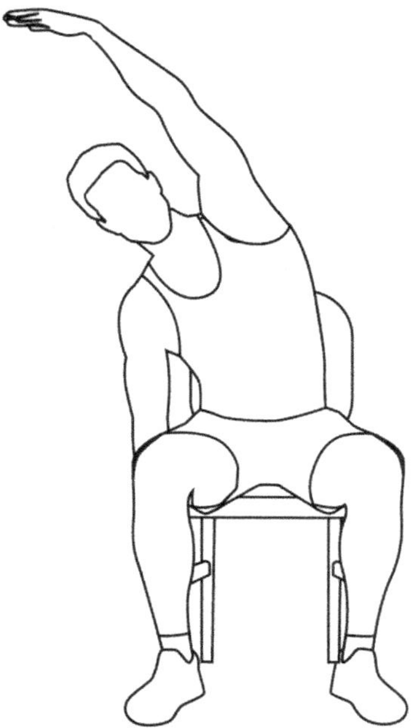

Side Stretch

1. Sit tall on your chair with feet placed flat on the floor, at about hip-width apart. Engage your core muscles to maintain a straight spine.
2. Raise one arm directly overhead, reaching towards the ceiling. Lengthen your side body by gently reaching your fingertips slightly higher with each inhale.
3. Slowly bend your torso sideways towards the unraised arm, reaching your other hand down towards the floor or the side of your chair seat (whichever feels comfortable). Avoid hunching your back – keep your spine long and your core engaged.
4. If comfortable, gently reach your raised hand even higher, feeling a deeper stretch along your side body. You can also soften your gaze and look up towards your raised hand for a more intense stretch in your neck and side torso.
5. Hold this gentle side stretch for several breaths, focusing on the lengthening sensation along your side. Breathe deeply with a steady rhythm throughout the hold.
6. Slowly return to center and repeat the same stretch on the other side. Breathe deeply and feel the stretch lengthen your opposite side body.

Chair Prayer Pose (Anjali Mudra)

The Chair Prayer Pose, also known as Anjali Mudra, brings a sense of inward focus and peace to your chair yoga practice. It promotes a gentle stretching in your shoulders and chest while fostering a feeling of centeredness. Here's how to find serenity in this pose:

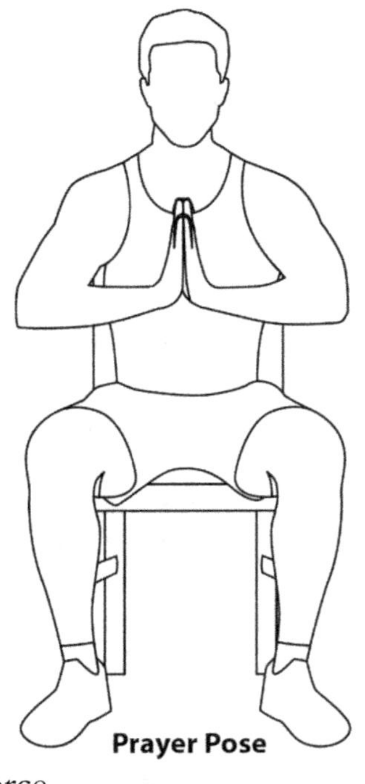

1. Begin by sitting tall on your chair with feet placed flat on the floor, at about hip-width apart. Lengthen your spine and let your shoulders relax.
2. Gently bring your palms together at your chest center, with your fingers pointing upwards. Keep your elbows soft and avoid pushing your hands together with force.
3. If comfortable, you can close your eyes softly to deepen your inward focus.
4. Take a few slow, deep breaths, feeling your abdomen and chest rise and fall gently. Focus on the connection between your breath and the gentle stretch in your chest and shoulders.
5. Hold this pose and take several breaths, allowing your body to settle into stillness. When you're ready, slowly release your hands and return them to your lap.

Chair Plank Pose (Phalakasana with Chair)

The Chair Plank Pose, also known as Phalasana with Chair in Sanskrit, is a fantastic way to build core strength and stability from the comfort of your chair. It engages your entire body, improving posture and balance. Here's how to find strength and control in this pose:

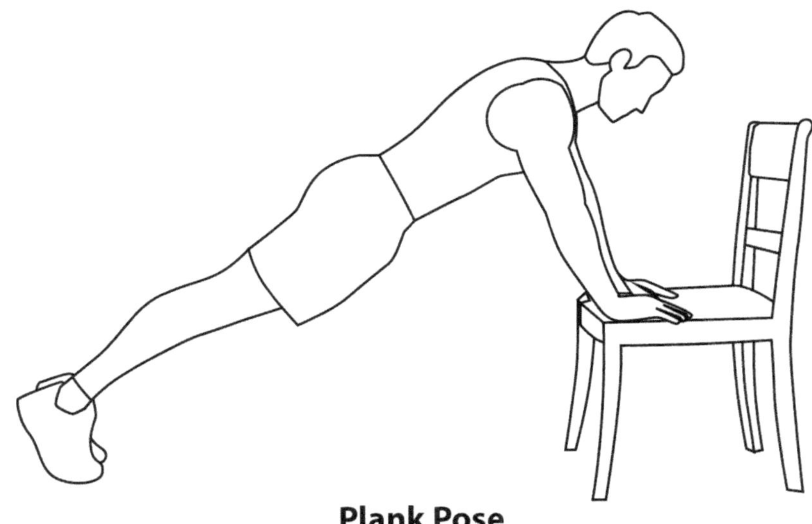

Plank Pose

1. Stand facing a sturdy chair, placing your hands shoulder-width apart on the chair seat.
2. Step back your feet one at a time until your body forms a straight line from your head to heels. Engage your core by drawing the belly button inwards towards your spine.
3. Maintain a long neck and spine by looking down slightly in front of your hands. Avoid letting your head hang or your back arch.
4. Press your heels firmly into the floor, keeping your legs straight and engaged.
5. Hold this plank position for several breaths, focusing on maintaining a strong core and a straight line with your body. Breathe deeply with a steady rhythm throughout the hold.

6. To release from the pose, slowly walk your feet back towards the chair until you are standing upright. Rest for a few breaths before repeating the pose if desired.

Chair Shoulder Stretch

Tight shoulders can lead to discomfort and restricted movement. This Chair Shoulder Stretch helps to improve shoulder mobility and release tension.

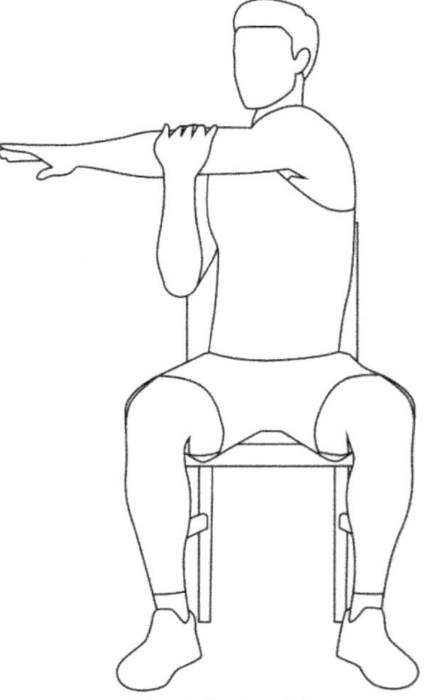

Shoulder Stretch

1. Sit comfortably on a chair with your feet flat on the ground and your spine tall, maintaining good posture.
2. Relax your shoulders down away from your ears, allowing your arms to hang naturally by your sides.
3. Inhale deeply, and as you exhale, reach across with your left hand and place it on your right elbow.
4. Gently pull your right arm towards your left side, feeling a stretch across the back of your right shoulder and upper arm.
5. Hold the stretch for a couple of breaths, maintaining gentle pressure to deepen the stretch without causing discomfort.
6. Inhale as you release your right arm back to the starting position.
7. Repeat the stretch on the opposite side by placing your right hand on your left elbow.
8. Gently guide your left arm towards your right side, feeling a stretch across the back of your left shoulder and upper arm.

9. Hold the stretch and take a few breaths, allowing the tension to release gradually.
10. Inhale as you bring your left arm back to the starting position.
11. For an additional stretch, clasp your hands behind your back, straightening your arms and gently lifting them away from your body.
12. Feel a stretch across the front of your shoulders and chest as you open your heart center.
13. Hold the stretch and take a few breaths, keeping your spine tall and your shoulders relaxed.
14. Release the clasp of your hands and return to a comfortable seated position.
15. Repeat the shoulder stretch sequence as needed, focusing on deep, mindful breaths to enhance relaxation and flexibility.

Chair Yoga Shoulder Rolls

Chair yoga shoulder rolls are a fantastic way to warm up your shoulders, improve their range of motion, and release any tension that might have built up throughout the day. Here's how to gently roll your shoulders in your chair:

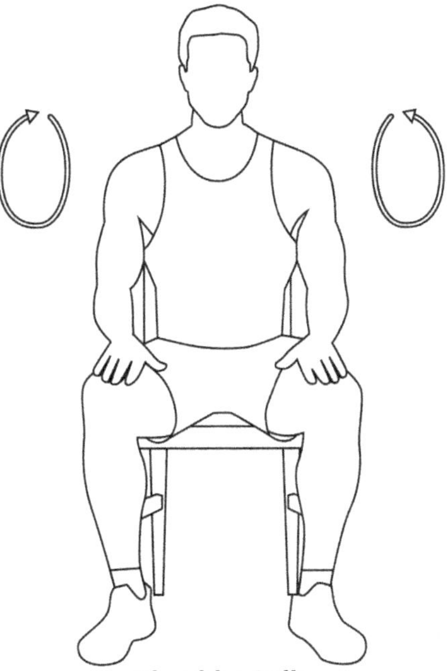

1. Begin by sitting tall in your chair with feet placed flat on the floor, at about hip-width apart. Engage your core muscles to maintain good posture.
2. Start by slowly shrugging your shoulders upwards towards your ears, as if

trying to reach them with your shoulder blades. Hold for a brief moment.

3. With your shoulders still raised, begin to roll them forward in a circular motion. Imagine you're drawing small circles with your shoulders. Make 5-10 small forward circles.
4. Once you've completed the forward rolls, reverse the direction and roll your shoulders backward in small circles for another 5-10 repetitions.
5. Continue rolling your shoulders forward and backward, focusing on a smooth and controlled movement. Breathe deeply with a steady rhythm throughout the exercise.

Chair Leg Extensions

Chair Leg Extensions are a simple yet effective way to improve leg strength and flexibility while seated. This exercise tones your quadriceps (muscles on the front of the thighs) and helps maintain healthy knee range of motion. Here's how to perform Chair Leg Extensions:

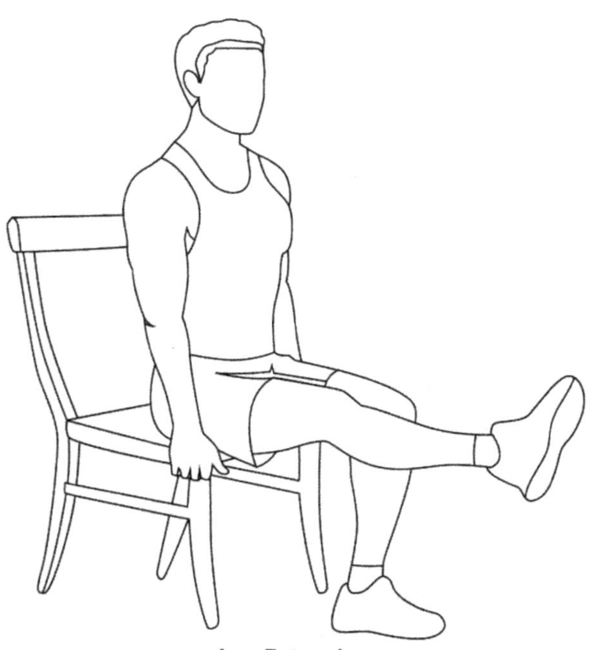

Leg Extensions

1. Begin by sitting upright on your chair with feet placed flat on the floor, at about hip-width apart. Engage your core by gently drawing your belly button inwards towards your spine.

2. Slowly stretch out one leg in front of you, keeping your heel
   on the floor if possible. If your heel doesn't comfortably
   reach the floor, point your toes and flex your foot.
3. Hold your extended leg straight for a few breaths, focusing
   on the gentle engagement in your quadriceps. Breathe deeply
   with a steady rhythm throughout the exercise.
4. Slowly lower your extended leg back down to the starting
   position. Repeat this extension movement with the other leg,
   completing the same number of holds and breaths.

Chair Butterfly Stretch

The Chair Butterfly Stretch targets
your inner thighs and groin muscles,
promoting flexibility and improving
range of motion in your hips. Here's
how to find a comfortable stretch in
this pose:

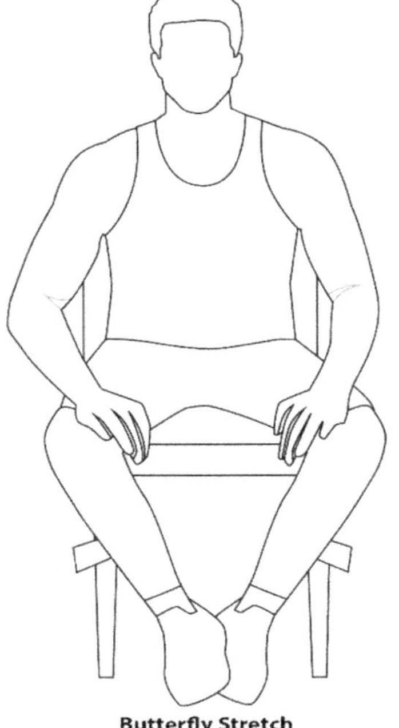

Butterfly Stretch

1. Begin by sitting on a sturdy
   chair with feet placed flat on
   the floor, at about hip-width
   apart. Engage your core and
   lengthen your spine by sitting
   tall.
2. Gently bring together the
   soles of your feet in front of
   you, creating a diamond shape
   with your knees pointing
   outwards.
3. Press your knees gently downwards towards the floor, feeling
   a stretch in your inner thighs. If comfortable, you can use
   your hands to press lightly on your knees to deepen the
   stretch, but avoid forcing it. Maintain a long, lengthened
   spine throughout the pose.

4. Inhale through your nose deeply and then exhale slowly through your mouth. Focus on your breath and feel the gentle tension in your inner thighs.

5. Hold this position for several breaths, allowing your body to relax and surrender to the stretch. When you're ready to release, slowly open your legs and return to the starting position.

Chair Yoga Wrist Stretches

Before diving into your chair yoga practice, it's important to prepare your wrists for movement. These gentle stretches help improve range of motion and flexibility, reducing the risk of strain. Here are a few effective wrist stretches to incorporate into your routine:

1. **Interlaced Stretch:** Sit comfortably on your chair with your back straight. Clasp your hands together in front of you, interlacing your fingers. Gently push your palms down, feeling a stretch in your forearms and your wrists. Hold the position for a few breaths, then relax and repeat with your fingers pointing upwards.

2. **Open Palm Stretch:** Extend one arm straight out in front of you, palm facing upwards. With your other hand, gently reach down and hold your outstretched fingers, applying a slight downward pressure. Feel a stretch along the top of your wrist and hand. Hold this position for a few breaths, then switch arms and repeat.

3. **Closed Fist Circles:** Make fists with both hands and stretch out your arms at shoulder height to the sides. Gently rotate your wrists in small circles, first forward for a few breaths, then backward for a few breaths. Focus on feeling the movement in your wrists rather than your elbows.

4. **Finger Flexion:** Extend both arms out in front of you, palms facing down. Spread your fingers wide and hold for some breaths. Then, gently clench your fingers into fists, hold for some breaths, and release. Repeat this sequence of

spreading and clenching a few times, feeling the movement in
your fingers and wrists.

Remember to breathe deeply and slowly throughout these stretches.
Pay attention to your body and avoid any movements that cause pain.

Chair Cactus Arms

The Seated Chair Cactus Arms
pose gently stretches and
strengthens your chest,
shoulders, and upper back
muscles. This pose is a great
way to improve your posture
and increase your range of
motion. Here's how to find
openness and strength in this
seated variation:

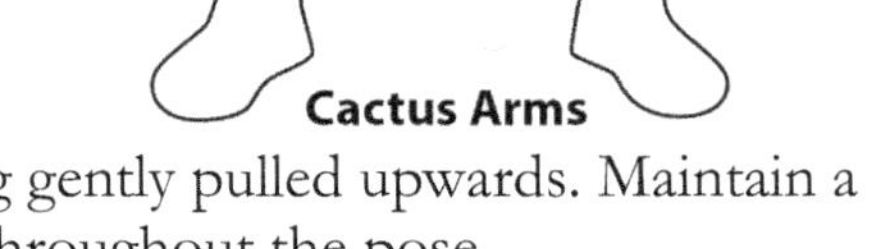

1. Begin by sitting
    comfortably on a sturdy
    chair with feet placed
    flat on the floor, at
    about hip-width apart.
    Lengthen your spine by
    imagining your head being gently pulled upwards. Maintain a
    tall and engaged posture throughout the pose.
2. Extend your two arms out to the sides, keeping them at
    shoulder height. Your palms can face forward or down,
    whichever feels more comfortable for you.
3. Bend your elbows at a 90-degree angle, forming a cactus-like
    shape with your arms. Imagine your upper arms reaching out
    to the sides while your forearms point upwards towards the
    ceiling.

4. Gently squeeze your core muscles, drawing your belly button inwards towards your spine. This helps to maintain proper posture and stability in your lower back.
5. Hold this pose and take several breaths, focusing on the gentle stretch across your chest and shoulders. Breathe deeply with a steady rhythm throughout the hold.
6. Slowly lower your arms back down to your sides, releasing any tension in your shoulders. Relax your core muscles and return to a comfortable seated position.

CHAPTER 5: INTERMEDIATE CHAIR YOGA POSES

As you build confidence and strength in your beginner chair yoga poses, you're ready to explore the intermediate level. These poses offer a deeper challenge, incorporating more balance work and stretches. They'll help you refine your yoga practice, improve coordination, and increase your range of motion. Don't hesitate to modify any pose to suit your abilities. It's important to pay attention to your body and gradually progress as you feel comfortable. Let's embark on this intermediate journey and discover new ways to challenge and invigorate yourself through chair yoga!

Chair Warrior I Pose (Virabhadrasana I)

The Chair Warrior I Pose, also known as Virabhadrasana I, is a powerful pose that builds leg strength, improves balance, and opens up the hips. With the chair as your support, you can explore this pose safely and effectively. Here's how to find your inner warrior:

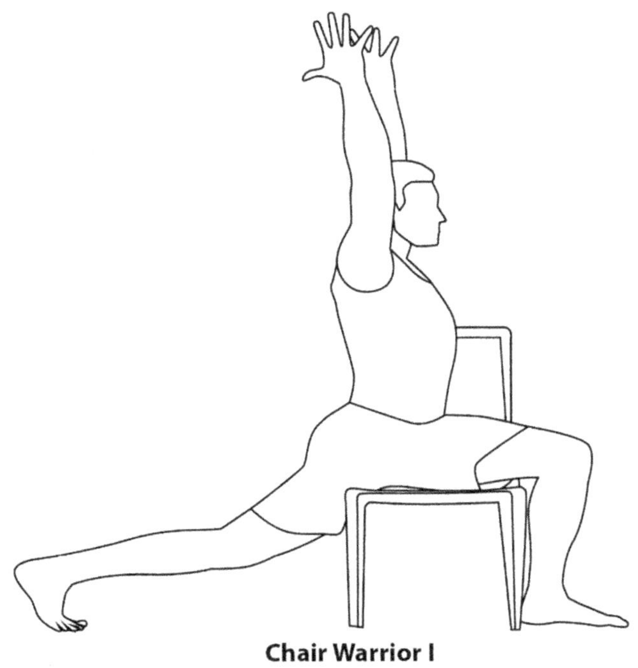

Chair Warrior I

43

1. Begin by sitting comfortably on the edge of a chair with both feet placed flat on the ground and your spine tall, maintaining good posture.
2. Slide your right foot back slightly, extending it behind you while keeping the toes pointing forward.
3. Ground your right heel firmly into the floor, maintaining stability.
4. Bend your left knee, ensuring it stays aligned over your left ankle, forming a 90-degree angle.
5. Keep your right leg straight and engaged, feeling a gentle stretch along the front of the right thigh and hip.
6. Inhale deeply, and as you exhale, engage your midsection muscles to stabilize your torso.
7. Raise your arms overhead, reaching towards the ceiling with your fingertips.
8. Keep your shoulders relaxed, maintaining length through your spine.
9. Gaze forward or slightly upward, finding a focal point to help you maintain balance and concentration.
10. Sink deeper into the stretch, feeling strength and stability in your legs and core.
11. Hold the pose and take several breaths, maintaining steady breathing and focusing on the sensation of grounding and expansion.
12. To release the pose, gently lower your arms back down by your sides and return your right foot to its starting position.
13. Repeat the sequence on the opposite side by sliding your left foot back, bending your right knee, and raising your arms overhead.
14. Ensure symmetry and balance between both sides of your body, adjusting as needed to maintain alignment and stability.
15. Practice the Chair Yoga Warrior I Pose regularly to strengthen the lower body, improve balance, and cultivate a sense of inner strength and focus.

Chair Warrior II Pose (Virabhadrasana II)

Chair Warrior II Pose, a variation of Virabhadrasana II, strengthens your legs and core while improving balance. Here's how to find power and stability in this seated pose:

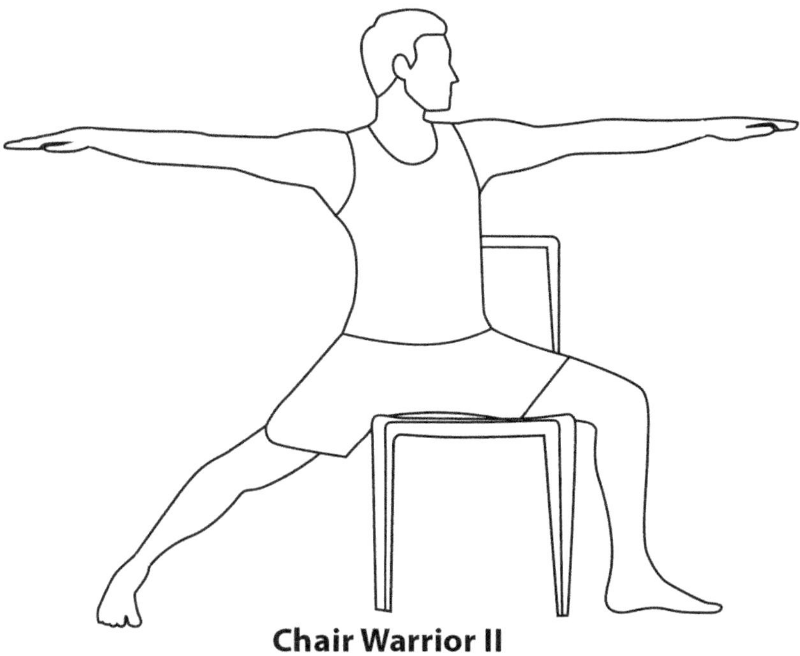

Chair Warrior II

1. Begin by sitting comfortably on the edge of a chair with both feet placed flat on the ground and your spine tall, maintaining good posture.
2. Slide back your right foot slightly, extending it behind you while keeping the toes pointing forward.
3. Ground your right heel firmly into the floor, maintaining stability.
4. Bend your left knee, ensuring it stays aligned over your left ankle, forming a 90-degree angle.
5. Keep your right leg straight and engaged, feeling a gentle stretch along the front of the right thigh and hip.
6. Inhale deeply, and as you exhale, engage your core muscles to stabilize your torso.

7. Gaze over your right fingertips, finding a focal point to help you maintain balance and concentration.
8. Keep your shoulders relaxed, maintaining length through your spine.
9. Sink deeper into the stretch, feeling strength and stability in your legs and core.
10. Hold the pose and take several breaths, maintaining steady breathing and focusing on the sensation of grounding and expansion.
11. To release the pose, gently straighten your right leg and lower your arms back down by your sides.
12. Rotate your right foot back to its starting position, aligning it with your left foot.
13. Repeat the sequence on the opposite side by turning your left foot out to the left side and bending your left knee.
14. Ensure symmetry and balance between both sides of your body, adjusting as needed to maintain alignment and stability.
15. Practice the Chair Yoga Warrior II Pose regularly to strengthen the lower body, improve balance, and cultivate a sense of inner strength and focus.

Chair Side Plank Pose

The Chair Side Plank Pose, a modification of chair plank pose, strengthens and tones your core and obliques while improving balance. By using the chair for support, you can achieve a side plank position even if you're new to yoga or have limited upper body strength. This pose lengthens your spine and improves stability in your shoulders and hips.

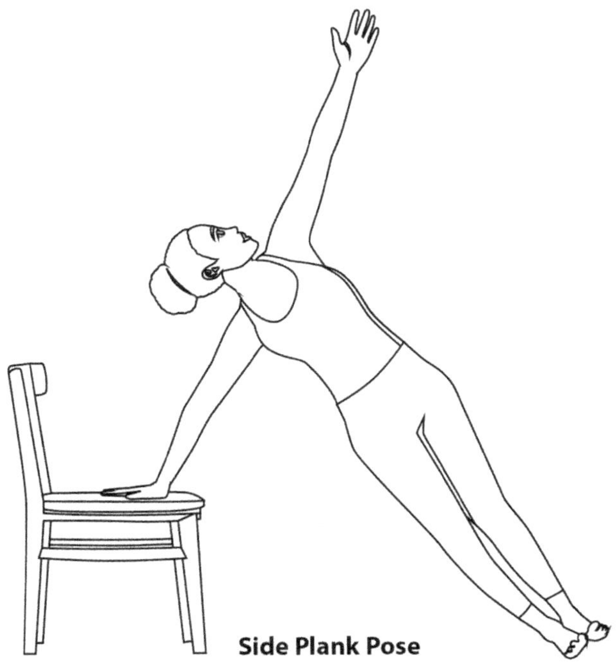

Side Plank Pose

1. Stand facing your sturdy chair, placing your hands shoulder-width apart on the chair seat.
2. Step back your feet one at a time until your body forms a straight line from your head to heels. Engage your core by drawing the belly button inwards towards your spine.
3. Maintain a long neck and spine by looking down slightly in front of your hands. Avoid letting your head hang or your back arch.
4. Press your heels firmly into the floor, keeping your legs straight and engaged.

5. Move your right hand to the center of the chair so that it can support your upper body alone then turn to face the left side lifting up your left hand straight up.
6. Maintain this position for a few breaths.
7. Repeat on the other side by supporting your body on the left hand, tuning to the right and lifting up the right hand.
8. To release from the pose, slowly walk your feet back towards the chair until you are standing upright. Rest for a few breaths before repeating the pose if desired.

Seated Reverse Plank

The Seated Reverse Plank strengthens your core muscles and improves upper body posture. Here's how to engage your core in this seated pose:

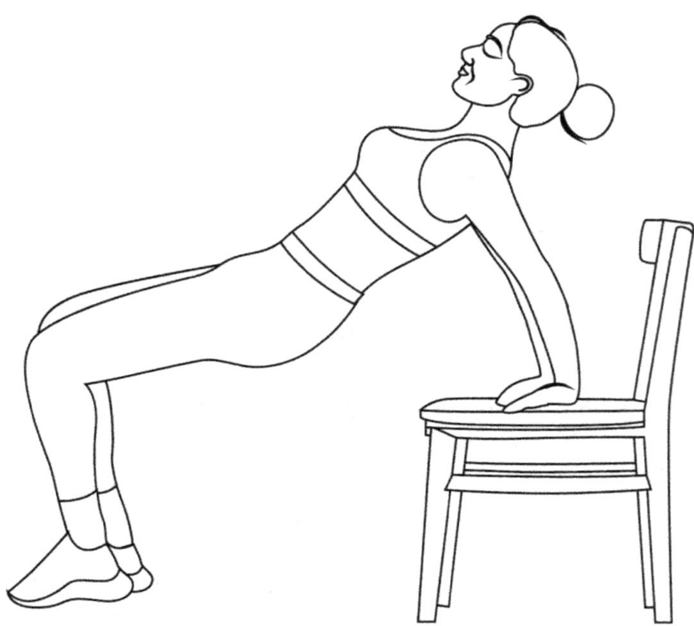

Reverse Plank

1. Sit tall at the edge of a sturdy chair with feet placed flat on the floor, at about hip-width apart. Draw your belly button inwards towards your spine to engage your core.
2. Gently lean back slightly, reaching your arms behind you. Find a comfortable distance where you can maintain good posture without straining your lower back.
3. Place both hands on the chair seat behind you, slightly wider than your shoulder-width apart. Your fingers should be pointing towards your body.
4. Press down firmly through your hands and engage your core to lift your hips slightly off the chair seat. Imagine your body forming a straight line from your shoulders to the knees.
5. Keep your neck long and your spine lengthened as you lift your hips. Avoid hunching your shoulders or rounding your back. You could also stretch out your legs.
6. Maintain this pose and take several breaths, focusing on the engagement in your core and the gentle stretch in your chest. Breathe deeply with a steady rhythm throughout the hold.
7. Slowly lower down your hips back to the chair seat, bringing your torso upright. Release your arms by your sides and relax your core muscles for a moment.
8. Repeat this pose for several repetitions to build core strength and improve your posture.

Seated Wide-Legged Forward Fold (Upavistha Konasana)

The Seated Wide-Legged Forward Fold, also known as Upavistha Konasana, stretches your inner thighs, hamstrings, and groin. It is simply the forward fold with legs opened wider. This pose can also improve flexibility in your lower back. Here's how to find a comfortable stretch in a chair:

1. Sit tall on your chair with feet placed flat on the floor, at about hip-width apart. Engage your core muscles by drawing your belly button inwards towards your spine.

2. Gently widen your legs as much as feels comfortable, keeping your feet placed flat on the floor. You can adjust the width based on your flexibility.
3. Inhale and lengthen your spine. As you exhale, hinge forward at your hips, keeping your back long and reaching your torso towards the floor. Imagine your tailbone lengthening towards the back of the chair.
4. Reach your hands forward towards the floor, shins, or chair seat, whichever is most comfortable. If reaching your hands down creates strain in your back, rest them gently on your thighs.
5. Keep your neck long and avoid straining. Look down towards the floor if comfortable, or keep your gaze forward.
6. Breathe deeply with a steady rhythm for several breaths, focusing on the gentle stretch in your inner thighs, hamstrings, and groin.
7. When ready to release, slowly engage your core muscles then lift your torso back up to starting position.

Chair Tree Pose (Vrksasana)

The Chair Tree Pose, also known as Vrksasana, helps develop balance and coordination. By utilizing the chair for support, you can experience the benefits of this pose in a safe and accessible way. Here's how to find your balance with the chair's assistance:

1. Begin by sitting comfortably on a chair with your feet flat on the ground and your spine tall. Find a steady and balanced position.
2. Ground down through your left foot and press it into the floor firmly to create a stable foundation.
3. Shift your weight slightly onto your left foot while keeping your right foot firmly planted on the ground.
4. Slowly lift your right foot off the ground, bending your right knee and bringing the sole of your right foot to rest on the inner left thigh or calf, depending on your flexibility and comfort level. Avoid placing the foot directly on the knee joint.
5. Find your balance by engaging your core muscles and focusing your gaze on a fixed point in front of you.
6. Bring your palms together in front of your chest in a prayer position, or if you prefer, extend your arms overhead with your palms facing each other.
7. Press your right foot firmly into the inner left calf or thigh while simultaneously pressing your left thigh or calf gently against your foot to create stability.

8. Keep your spine tall and your shoulders relaxed, finding a sense of length and openness through the crown of your head.
9. Engage your core muscles so as to help you maintain balance and stability in the pose.
10. Take a couple of deep breaths, feeling rooted and grounded through your standing leg while reaching upward through your arms.
11. If you feel steady, you can experiment with swaying gently from side to side, mimicking the movement of a tree in the breeze.
12. Hold the pose and take several breaths, enjoying the sensation of being both grounded and expansive.
13. To release the pose, slowly lower your right foot back to the ground and return to a seated position on the chair.
14. Take a little moment to notice how you feel after practicing Chair Yoga Tree Pose, observing any changes in your balance, posture, or energy levels.
15. If you like, you can repeat the pose on the opposite side, balancing on your right foot and placing your left foot on your inner right thigh or calf.

Chair High Lunge (Ashwa Sanchalanasana)

The Chair High Lunge, a variation of Ashwa Sanchalanasana, strengthens your quads, improves balance, and offers a gentle stretch for your hamstrings. Here's how to find power and flexibility in this lunge:

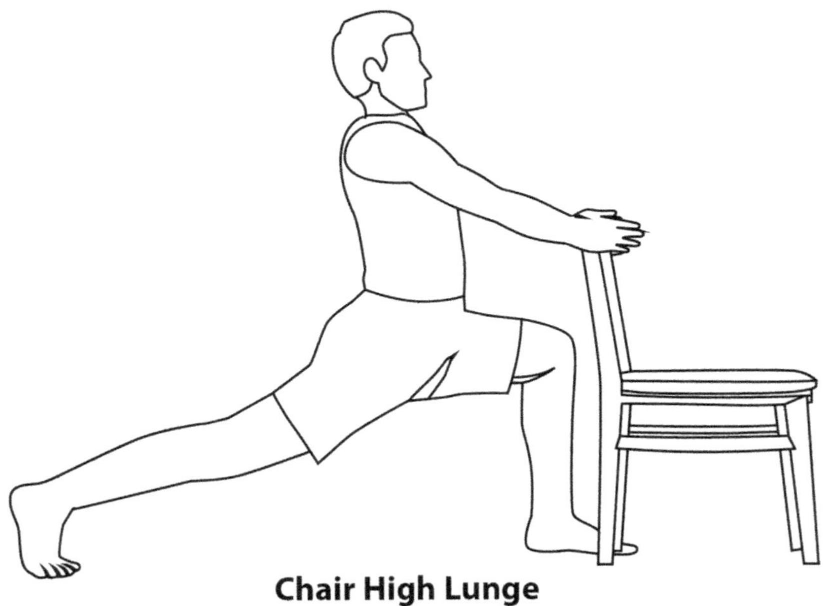

Chair High Lunge

1. Stand beside a sturdy chair, holding onto the back of your chair for support with one hand.
2. Step one leg back, keeping your front foot flat on the floor. Bend your front knee at a 90-degree angle, ensuring your front knee stays directly over your ankle.
3. Engage your core and lengthen your spine, keeping your back straight and avoiding hunching.
4. Reach your torso forward slightly, keeping your hips square and back long. You can rest your other hand on your front thigh for added balance.
5. Hold this pose and take several breaths, focusing on the sensation of strength in your front leg and a gentle stretch in

your back leg's hamstring. Breathe deeply with a steady rhythm throughout the hold.

6. Slowly push back up to the position you started from, engaging your front leg muscle. Repeat the same pose on the other side, stepping back with your opposite leg and bending your standing knee.

Seated Hamstring Stretch

The Seated Hamstring Stretch gently lengthens the muscles on the back of your thighs, the hamstrings, improving flexibility and reducing tightness. Here's how to find a comfortable stretch in this chair-supported pose:

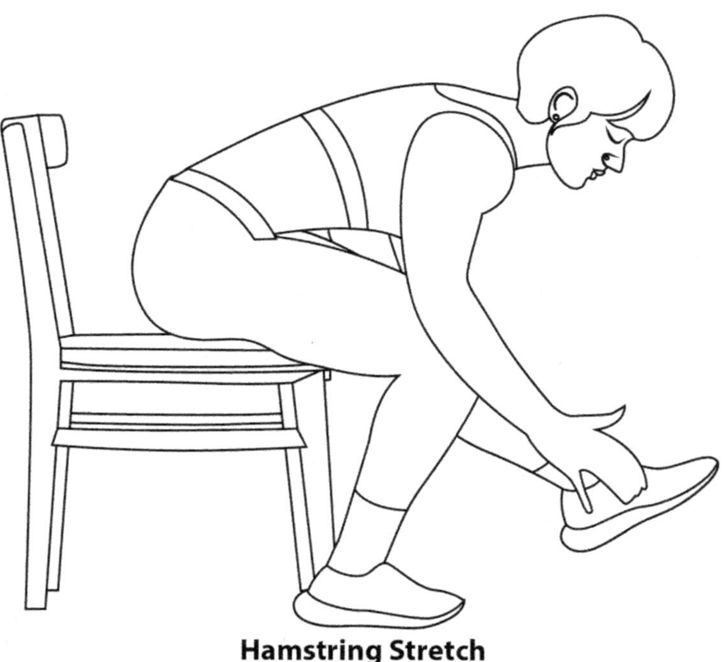

Hamstring Stretch

1. Begin by sitting tall on your chair with both feet placed flat on the floor, hip-width apart. Draw your belly button inwards towards your spine to engage your core.

2. Extend one leg out straight in front of you, keeping the heel on the floor. Point your toes upwards and flex your foot if needed.

3. Inhale and gently hinge forward from your hips, reaching your torso towards your extended leg. Keep your back long and try not to round your spine. Imagine lengthening your spine with each inhale.

4. You can reach for your toes or the top of your foot with both hands. If this is uncomfortable, gently loop a strap or yoga belt around the arch of your extended foot and hold onto the ends with both hands. This will assist you in reaching further.

5. As you reach or hold onto your leg, keep your back long and avoid hunching forward. You should feel a gentle stretch in the back of your extended leg.

6. Breathe deeply and hold this stretch for several breaths, allowing your hamstrings to gradually lengthen. Focus on the sensation of the stretch and avoid pushing yourself to the point of pain.

7. Inhale and slowly return to the starting position. Repeat the stretch on the other side, extending your opposite leg and reaching towards your foot.

Chair Camel Pose

Chair Camel Pose, while not as intense as the traditional Camel Pose done on the floor, offers a taste of its benefits in a safe and supported way. By gently opening your chest and stretching the front of your body, this pose can help to improve posture, increase flexibility in the spine and shoulders, and even stimulate your digestive system. It's a great addition to your chair yoga routine for a touch of gentle backbending and an overall sense of openness.

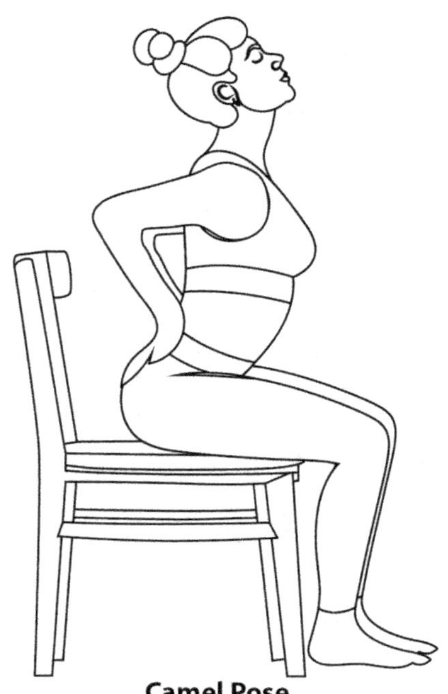

Camel Pose

1. Sit comfortably on a chair with your feet flat on the ground and your spine tall, maintaining good posture.
2. Place both hands on your lower back, fingertips pointing downward, with your palms resting on the back of the chair.
3. Inhale deeply, lengthening through your spine, and gently arch your back, drawing your chest forward and upward.
4. Press your hips forward slightly, allowing your pelvis to tilt forward while keeping your feet grounded.
5. Lift your heart towards the ceiling, opening up through the front of your body.
6. Keep your shoulders relaxed, avoiding any tension in the neck or upper back.
7. Hold the pose for a couple of breaths, feeling a stretch across the front of your chest and abdomen.
8. If comfortable, you can tilt your head back slightly, gazing upwards without straining the neck.
9. Breathe deeply and evenly, allowing the breath to support the opening and expansion of your chest.

10. To deepen the stretch, you can gently press your hands into your lower back, encouraging further arching of the spine.

11. Be mindful not to overextend or strain, listening to your body and finding a position that feels comfortable yet challenging.

12. Hold the Seated Camel Pose for several breaths, enjoying the sensation of openness and expansion in the front body.

13. To release the pose, exhale slowly and return to an upright seated position, bringing your hands back to your lap.

14. Take a little moment to notice how you feel after practicing the Seated Camel Pose, observing any changes in your posture, breath, or sense of openness.

15. Repeat the pose as desired, focusing on maintaining a smooth and steady breath while exploring the stretch and expansion of the front body.

Chair Boat Pose (Navasana Variation)

Chair Boat Pose, a variation of Navasana, strengthens and tones your core muscles while improving your balance. Here's how to engage your core and find stability in this seated pose:

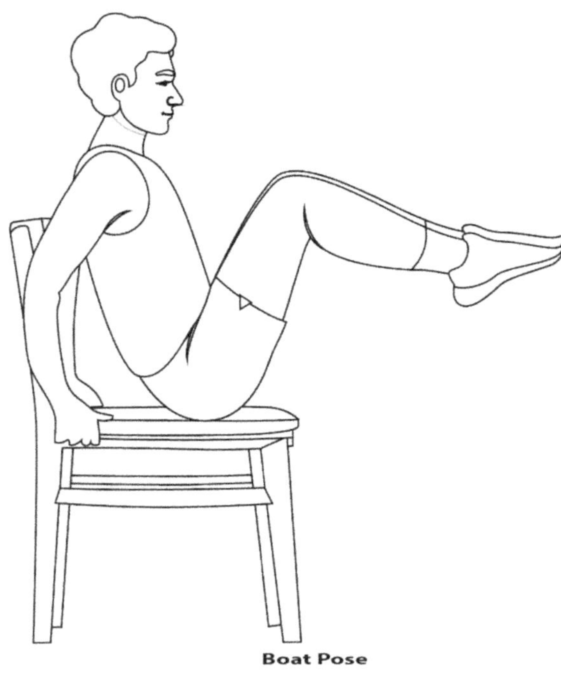

1. Begin by sitting on the front edge of your chair with feet

placed flat on the floor, at about hip-width apart. Draw your belly button inwards towards your spine to engage your core and lengthen your spine upwards.

2. Slowly lean back slightly, keeping your back straight and engaging your core muscles to maintain your balance. You can use your hands to hold the sides of the chair seat for additional support if needed.

3. As you continue to engage your core, slowly lift your feet off the floor, keeping your legs extended or slightly bent at the knees.

4. Focus on maintaining a straight spine and a long neck. If lifting both legs is challenging, you can start by lifting one leg at a time.

5. Hold this pose and take several breaths, focusing on the engagement in your core and the feeling of balance. Breathe deeply with a steady rhythm throughout the hold.

6. Slowly lower your feet down back to the floor, one at a time or both together, while maintaining good posture. You can repeat this pose for several sets of breaths to enhance the core workout.

Chair Seated Eagle Pose (Garudasana)

Chair Seated Eagle Pose, a variation of Garudasana, challenges your balance and improves coordination in the upper body. Here's how to explore this pose from the comfort of your chair:

1. Begin by sitting tall on your chair with feet placed flat on the floor, at about hip-width apart. Engage your core muscles for stability.
2. Lift one foot and cross it over your other ankle, aiming to wrap the foot around your calf if possible. For added comfort, you can rest the sole of your lifted foot on your other shin.
3. Extend your forearms out to the front. Bend your elbows, bringing your forearms parallel to the floor.
4. Weave your forearms by bringing one arm underneath the other. If comfortable, try to clasp your hands together with palms facing inwards. Alternatively, you can rest the back of one hand on the back of the other.
5. Gently lift your elbows towards the ceiling, lengthening your spine and maintaining an upright posture. Focus on keeping your shoulders relaxed.
6. Maintain this pose and take several breaths, focusing on your balance and the connection between your arms. Breathe deeply with a steady rhythm throughout the hold.
7. Slowly unwind your arms and release your crossed legs back to the starting position. Repeat the same pose on the other

Eagle Pose

side, crossing your opposite ankle over your calf and weaving your arms in the opposite direction.

Chair Pigeon Pose (Eka Pada Rajakapotasana)

The Chair Pigeon Pose, also known as Eka Pada Rajakapotasana, targets your hips and glutes, promoting flexibility and relieving tension. This pose is done while seated in your chair, thereby making it accessible for various fitness levels.

Here's how to find a gentle stretch in your hips with the Chair Pigeon Pose:

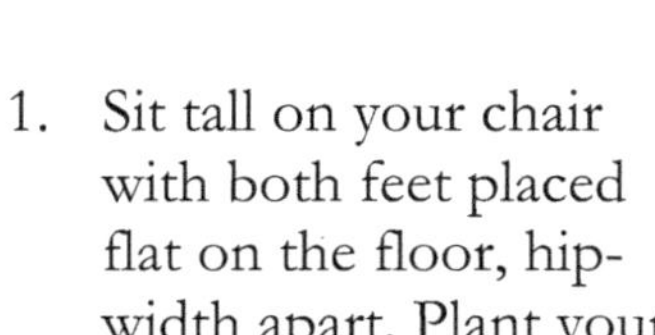

Pigeon Pose

1. Sit tall on your chair with both feet placed flat on the floor, hip-width apart. Plant your right foot firmly on the ground and lift the left foot off the floor.
2. Cross your left ankle over the right knee, creating a figure-four shape with your legs. Flex the foot of the crossed leg for stability.
3. Flex your left foot to protect your ankle and knee joints, ensuring your left knee points directly away from your body. Keep your spine tall and your chest lifted, maintaining good posture throughout the pose.
4. To deepen the stretch, Lift up your hands, hinge at the hips and lean your torso forward, reaching towards your extended leg. Keep your back long and avoid hunching. You can rest

your forearms on your chair seat or the floor for support, depending on your flexibility.

5. Hold this pose and take several breaths, focusing on the gentle stretch in your hips and buttocks. Breathe deeply with a steady rhythm throughout the hold.

6. Slowly return to the starting position and repeat the same pose on the other side, crossing your opposite ankle over your thigh and extending the other leg back.

CHAPTER 6: ADVANCED CHAIR YOGA POSES

Having mastered the foundational poses of chair yoga, you might be feeling a surge of confidence and a desire to explore more challenging movements. This section dives into the realm of advanced chair yoga poses. These postures will test your balance, flexibility, and core strength, while offering a deeper mind-body connection. Remember, it's crucial to pay attention to your body and prioritize safety over pushing your limits. If a pose feels uncomfortable, don't hesitate to modify it or gently come out of it. With dedication and a playful spirit, you'll be surprised by the progress you can make in your advanced chair yoga practice!

Chair Extended Side Angle Pose (Utthita Parsvakonasana) (Modification)

The Chair Extended Side Angle Pose, a variation of Utthita Parsvakonasana, stretches and strengthens your legs, hips, and core while improving balance. Here's how to find an open and invigorating side stretch chair support:

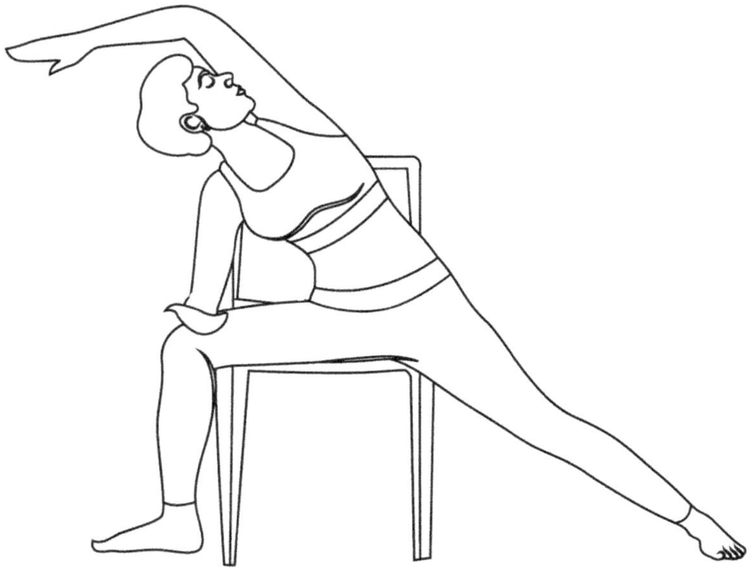

Extended Side Angle Pose

1. Begin by sitting sideways on a sturdy chair. Position your body so that your right hip and buttock are closer to the chair back.
2. Extend your right leg straight out to the side, keeping your heel flat on the floor. Flex your foot for added stability.
3. Bend your left knee at a 90-degree angle, placing your left foot flat on the floor directly under your left knee. Align your left ankle directly beneath your left hip for proper posture.

4. Reach your left arm overhead, extending your fingertips towards the ceiling. Imagine lengthening your spine as you reach upwards.
5. If comfortable, you can gently twist your torso to the right, gazing upwards towards your extended left arm. Keep your hips facing forward as much as possible during the twist.
6. Maintain this pose and take several breaths, feeling the stretch along the side of your body and the activation of your core muscles. Breathe deeply with a steady rhythm throughout the hold.
7. Slowly unwind any twist, lower your left arm down, and bring your right leg back to starting position. Repeat the same on the other side, extending your left leg out straight and reaching your right arm overhead.

Chair-Supported Crane Pose With Blocks (Bakasana Variation)

Chair-Supported Crane Pose with blocks offers a playful and accessible way to work towards the traditional Crane Pose. By utilizing blocks and a chair, you'll gain the confidence and support needed to explore balancing on your forearms.

Preparation:

- Two yoga blocks (or sturdy books)
- A sturdy chair

Here's how to find your balance in this pose:

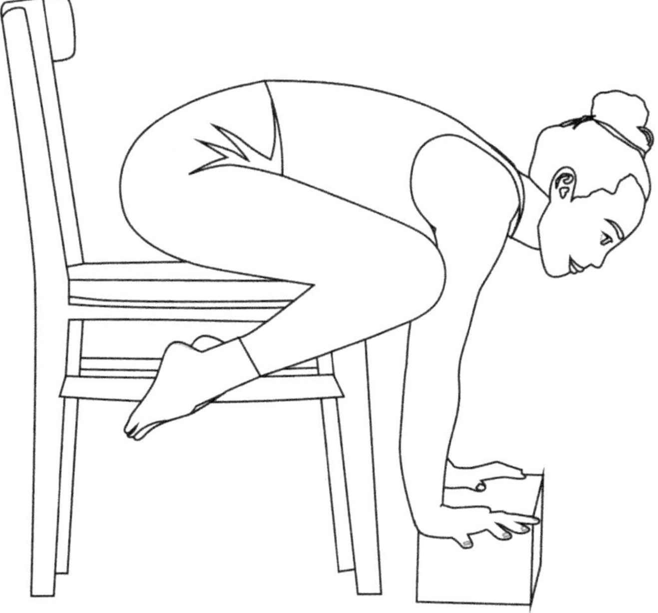

Supported Crane Pose

1. Place the blocks shoulder-width apart in front of your chair, about a foot away. You can adjust the block height based on

your comfort level – start higher for more support and gradually lower them as you progress.

2. Sit on the chair with feet placed flat on the floor, at about hip-width apart. Draw your belly button inwards to engage your core.
3. Place your hands flat on the yoga blocks, fingers spread wide. Lean forward from your hips, keeping your back straight and core engaged.
4. Maintain a forward gaze, looking slightly beyond your fingertips for better balance.
5. As you engage your core further, gently lift your hips and knees off the chair, aiming to bring your shins towards your chest.
6. Hold this pose and take several breaths, focusing on maintaining a stable and comfortable position on your forearms.
7. If you feel comfortable and balanced, you can try lifting one foot off the floor and extending it behind you. Hold the position for a few breaths before slowly lowering your foot and returning to the starting position.
8. Gently lower your hips and knees back down to sit on the chair. Take a couple of deep breaths to rest before repeating the pose.

Remember: This pose requires balance and core strength. If you feel unstable, it's perfectly fine to keep your knees bent or hold the pose for shorter durations.

Chair-Supported Wheel Pose (Urdhva Dhanurasana)

Chair-Supported Wheel Pose, a variation of Urdhva Dhanurasana, offers a safe and accessible way to experience a gentle backbend using a chair and props. This pose strengthens your core, improves flexibility, and opens up your chest.

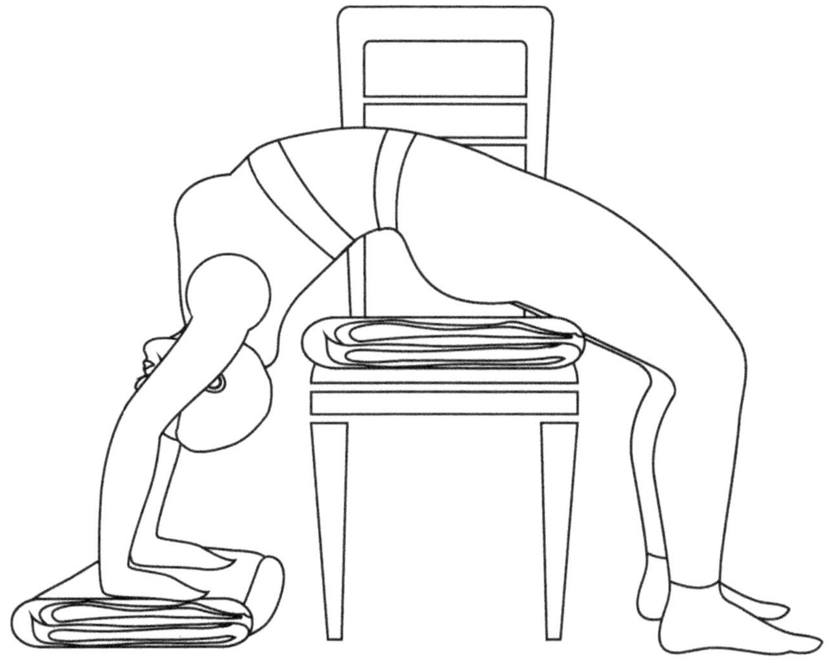

Supported Wheel Pose

1. Place a blanket on your chair and a pillow on one side of it.
2. Sit sideways on the chair on the opposite side to the pillow.
3. Hold the back of the chair to provide support then lean backwards until your body is draped on the chair and your feet resting on the floor. You can rest your head on the pillow but don't put your weight on your neck.
4. Stretch out your hands over your head towards the floor with palms facing your feet. Release any tension in shoulders and neck.

5. If comfortable, gently arch your back, pressing your chest forward and lifting your chin slightly. Remember: Don't force the backbend.
6. Maintain this pose and take several breaths, focusing on the gentle stretch in your chest and the strength in your core and legs. Breathe deeply with a steady rhythm throughout the hold.
7. To come out of this pose, slowly raise your hands to grab the back or seat of the chair, press your heels into the ground for support and then pull yourself to the sitting position.

Chair Triceps Dips

Chair Triceps Dips target your triceps, the muscles on the backside of your upper arms. This pose strengthens and defines these muscles, improving upper body strength and stability. Here's how to effectively perform Seated Chair Triceps Dips:

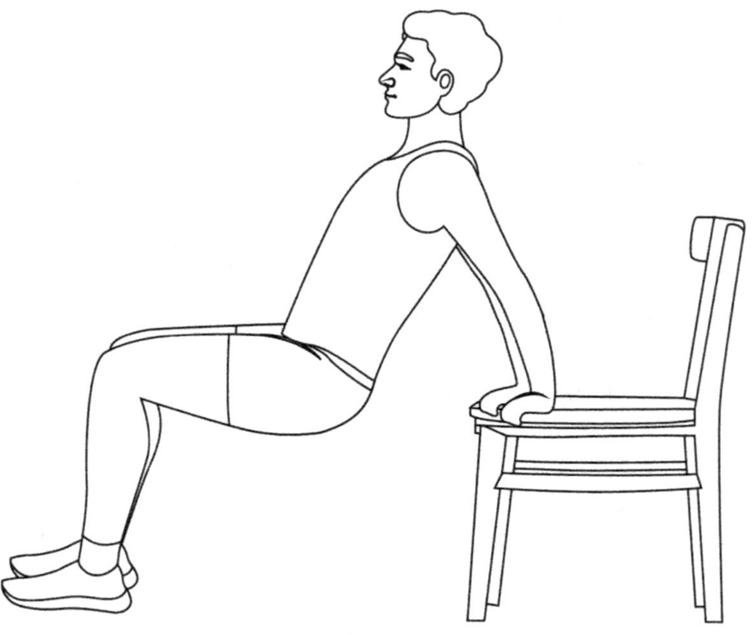

Triceps Dips

1. Sit on the edge of your chair with feet placed flat on the floor, at about hip-width apart.
2. Place your hands shoulder-width apart on the chair beside your hips, fingers pointing forward.
3. Engage your core and gently lift your hips off the chair, straightening your legs slightly. Avoid locking your knees.
4. Bend your elbows, lowering your body down towards the floor until your elbows reach a 90-degree angle. Keep your back close to the chair and your core engaged.
5. Press down firmly through your palms and straighten your elbows to return to your starting position.
6. Complete several repetitions of this dip, focusing on controlled movements and deep breaths. Inhale as you lower yourself down and exhale as you are pushing back up.

Chair Revolved Side Stretch With Arm Reach (Revolved Triangle Pose With Chair)

This pose is a modification of the Chair Revolved Triangle Pose that offers a slightly gentler variation with a focus on opening the side of your body. Here's how to find a comfortable twist and reach:

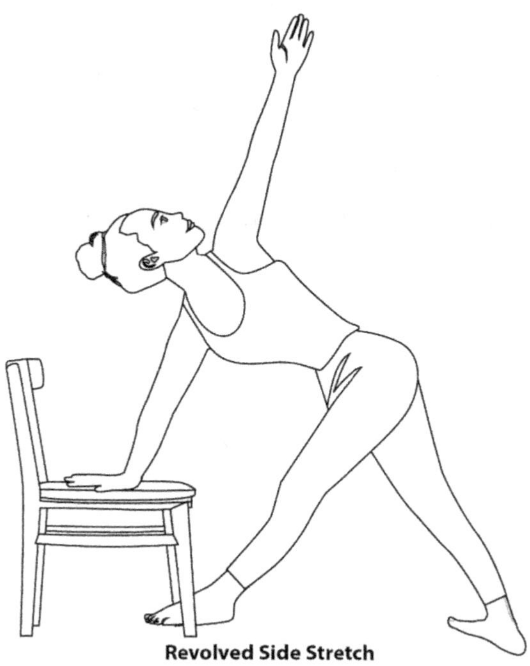

Revolved Side Stretch

1. Stand upright with your feet hip-width apart, facing a sturdy chair. Position your right leg closest to the chair for added stability.
2. Extend your left arm and place your hand on the chair seat or back, depending on what feels most comfortable and supportive.
3. Breathe in deeply. As you are inhaling, raise your right arm overhead, reaching your fingertips towards the ceiling. Imagine stretching your chest upwards lengthen your spine.
4. Gently squeeze your shoulder blades together, feeling a deeper engagement in your upper back muscles.

5. As you exhale, slowly lower your right arm back down to rest on the chair seat or back. Maintain a little bend in your right knee for stability throughout the movement.
6. Repeat this reaching motion with your right arm for 8 breaths, inhaling as you reach up and exhaling as you lower your arm down. Focus on a smooth, rhythmic flow with your breath and movement.
7. After completing 8 repetitions, release your right arm and come back to standing upright. Repeat the entire sequence on the other side, bringing your left leg closer to the chair and reaching your left arm overhead.

Chair Downward-Facing Dog Pose (Adho Mukha Svanasana) (Modification)

The Chair Downward-Facing Dog Pose, a variation of Adho Mukha Svanasana, offers a gentle way to experience the benefits of the classic Downward-Facing Dog while using a chair for support. This pose stretches your hamstrings, strengthens your arms and shoulders, and improves circulation. Here's how to find length and stability in this pose:

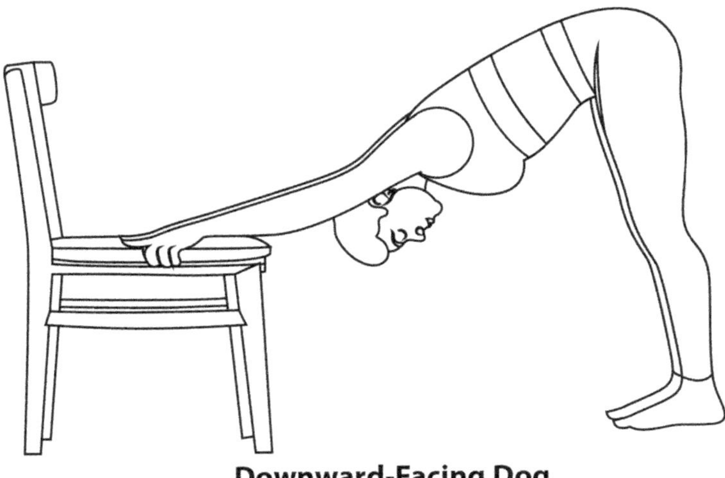

Downward-Facing Dog

1. Stand tall in front of a sturdy chair, with your feet about hip-width apart. Draw your belly button inwards towards your spine to engage your core muscles.
2. Take a step back with both feet, keeping your heels flat on the floor. As you step back, hinge at the hips and lengthen your spine, reaching your torso forward towards the chair.
3. Place your hands shoulder-width apart on the chair seat or back, depending on what feels comfortable and provides the most support.
4. Straighten out your arms as much as you can without locking your elbows. Concentrate on lengthening your spine and pushing your hips back towards the wall behind you.
5. Keep your knees at a slight bend, engaging your leg muscles to avoid placing your entire weight on your arms. Imagine pressing your heels firmly into the floor, even if they don't reach the ground.
6. Keep your neck long and in line with your spine. Avoid looking up or down excessively.
7. Hold this pose and take several breaths, focusing on the stretch in your hamstrings and the feeling of length in your spine. Breathe deeply with a steady rhythm throughout the hold.
8. Slowly push yourself back up to standing by straightening your legs and engaging your core muscles. Take a moment to rest in standing before repeating the pose if desired.

Chair Half Moon Pose (Ardha Chandrasana) (Modification)

The Chair Half Moon Pose, a variation of Ardha Chandrasana, challenges your balance while offering the chair support for stability. This pose strengthens your legs and core while improving proprioception (body awareness).

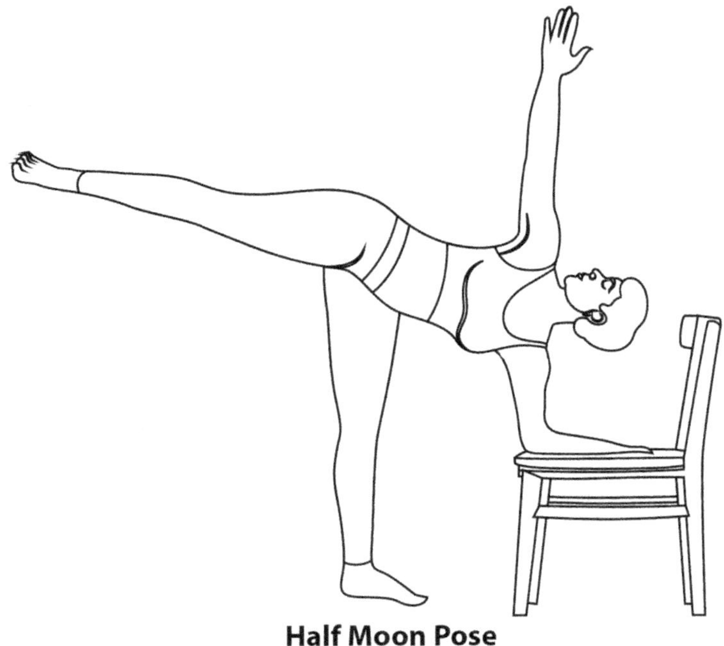

Half Moon Pose

1. Stand beside a sturdy chair with your feet hip-width apart. Draw your belly button inwards towards your spine to engage your core.
2. Extend the right arm overhead, reaching your fingertips towards the ceiling. Place your left hand on the chair back for support. You may also place it on the seat of the chair.
3. Shift your bodyweight onto your right leg, keeping your right foot flat on the floor. As you exhale, gently lift your left leg off the ground, extending it straight out behind you. Maintain a little bend in your standing right knee.

4. Look upwards towards your extended right arm, keeping your neck long. Imagine lengthening your entire spine from your tailbone to your head.

5. Hold this pose and take several breaths, focusing on maintaining balance and stability with the support of the chair. Breathe deeply and evenly throughout the hold.

6. Keep your midsection muscles engaged to help prevent your lower back from arching. If you feel any strain in your lower back, adjust the position of your lifted leg or come back to standing.

7. Slowly lower your left leg back down to the floor, returning to the starting position. Repeat the same on the other side, stretching your left arm overhead and placing your right hand on the chair back or seat for support.

Chair Sun Salutation Sequence

The Chair Sun Salutation Sequence, a modification of the traditional Sun Salutation, offers a dynamic and energizing way to move your body from a seated position. By using the chair for support, you can experience the benefits of this flowing sequence without putting straining your joints. Let's link breath with movement in this invigorating practice:

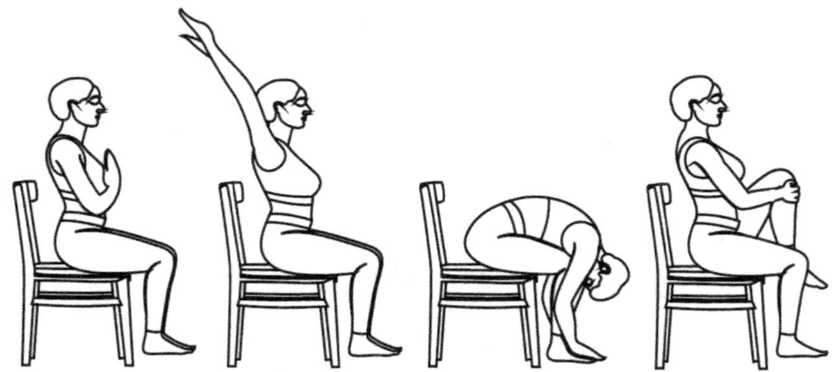

Sun Salutation Sequence

74

1. **Seated Mountain Pose (Tadasana):** Begin by sitting tall on your chair with feet placed flat on the floor, at about hip-width apart. Put hands together in front of your chest, draw your belly button inwards towards your spine to engage your core and lengthen your spine, imagining your head being gently pulled upwards. Take a couple of deep breaths to center yourself.

2. **Inhale and Reach Up (Hastalambasana):** Inhale deeply and raise both arms overhead, stretching your fingertips towards the ceiling. Open your chest and feel your shoulder blades gently squeezing together. Hold for a moment, feeling the stretch in your sides and upper back.

3. **Exhale and Fold Forward (Uttanasana):** As you exhale, hinge at the hips and fold your torso forward, keeping your back long. Reach your hands towards your shins or the floor, depending on your flexibility. Let your head hang heavy and feel a gentle stretch in your hamstrings and the lower back. Hold for some breaths.

4. **Inhale, raise your torso and raise a knee (Ardha Pavan Muktasana):** Raise your torso back to sitting position then lift up one of your knees towards your chest holding it with your palms. Exhale and bring your forehead down close to the knee.

5. **Exhale** as you returned the raised foot back to the floor.

6. **Inhale and Reach Up (Hastalambasana):** Inhale and raise both arms overhead again, stretching your fingertips towards the ceiling. Open your chest and feel your shoulder blades gently squeezing together. Hold for an instant, feeling the stretch in your sides and upper back.

7. **Exhale and Return to Seated (Tadasana):** Exhale and slowly bring your arms back down to your sides. Return to a seated position on your chair, with your feet placed flat on the floor and your spine lengthened. Take a couple of deep breaths to rest and integrate the movement.

8. **Repeat on the Other Side:** Repeat this entire sequence, starting with Step 2, but this time stepping your left leg back in Step 6. Continue to alternate sides with each repetition.

Remember: Pay attention to your body and modify the poses as needed. Breathe deeply with a steady rhythm throughout the flow to enhance your experience.

Chair Squats

Chair squats are a fantastic way to build strength and stability in your legs while using the chair for support. This simple yet effective exercise targets your quads, hamstrings, and glutes. Here's how to perform chair squats with proper form:

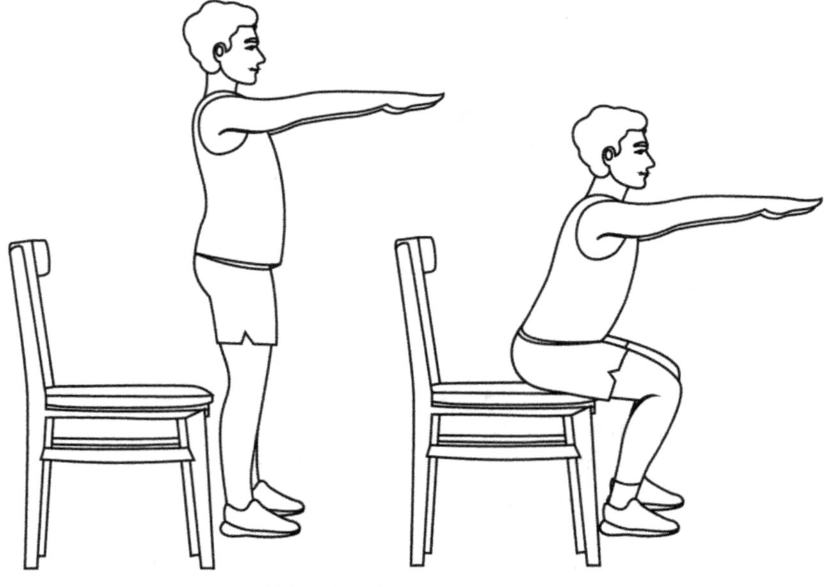

Chair Squats

1. Begin by standing in front of your chair with your feet hip-width apart and toes pointed slightly outward. Maintain a tall posture with your shoulders relaxed and your core engaged.
2. For added balance, you can extend your arms straight out in front of you at shoulder height.
3. Inhale and begin to lower yourself down as if you're going to sit in the chair. Keep your back straight and your core

engaged throughout the movement. Imagine pushing your hips back and down, rather than bending directly at your knees.

4. As you lower yourself, bend your knees at a 90-degree angle, keeping your knees aligned with your ankles. Avoid letting your knees cave inwards.

5. Ideally, aim to gently tap your buttocks on the chair seat or hover slightly above it without actually sitting down.

6. Exhale as you press down through your heels to push yourself back up to your starting position. Maintain a controlled movement throughout the squat.

7. Repeat this squat motion for a desired number of repetitions, typically 8-12 repetitions. Focus on maintaining proper form and breathing deeply throughout your set.

8. Take a short rest after completing a set of squats, then repeat the exercise for additional sets if desired. You can gradually increase the number of repetitions over time as your strength improves.

Chair Warrior III Pose (Virabhadrasana III) (Modification)

The Chair Warrior III Pose, inspired by Virabhadrasana III, challenges your balance and strengthens your legs and core. With the chair support, you can explore this pose safely and build confidence. Here's how to find your warrior within:

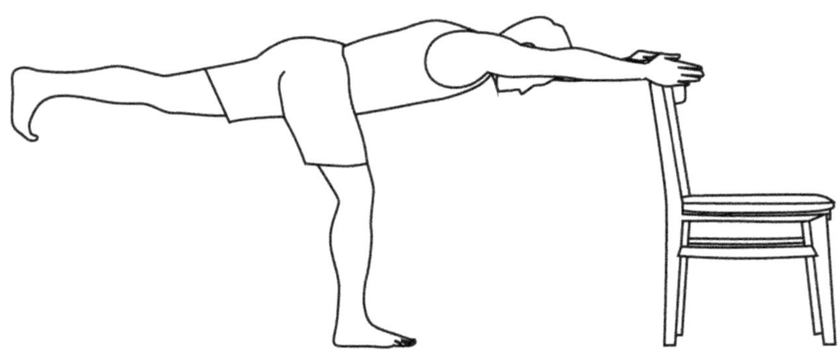

Chair Warrior III

1. Stand beside a sturdy chair with your feet hip-width apart.
    Engage your core muscles by drawing your belly button
    inwards towards your spine.
2. Shift your weight onto your right leg, keeping your right foot
    firmly planted on the floor.
3. Extend your left leg straight back behind you, keeping your
    heel lifted off the floor. Flex your left foot for added stability.
4. Reach your arms straight up overhead, lengthening your spine
    and gazing upwards towards your fingertips. Imagine
    reaching for the ceiling with your fingertips.
5. Keep a straight back and avoid arching your lower back.
    Engage your core muscles to maintain a neutral spine all
    through the pose.
6. Hold this Warrior III pose for several breaths, focusing on
    the sensation of balance and strength in your standing leg and
    core. Breathe deeply with a steady rhythm throughout the
    hold.
7. Slowly lower your extended leg back down to the floor and
    return to standing upright on both feet. Repeat the same on
    the other side, extending your right leg back and reaching
    your arms overhead.

Chair Yoga Bridge Pose (Setubandha Sarvangasana with Chair)

The Yoga Bridge Pose with a chair provides an excellent stretch for the chest, shoulders, and hips, while also strengthening the legs and core muscles. Practice mindfully and enjoy the benefits of this rejuvenating posture.

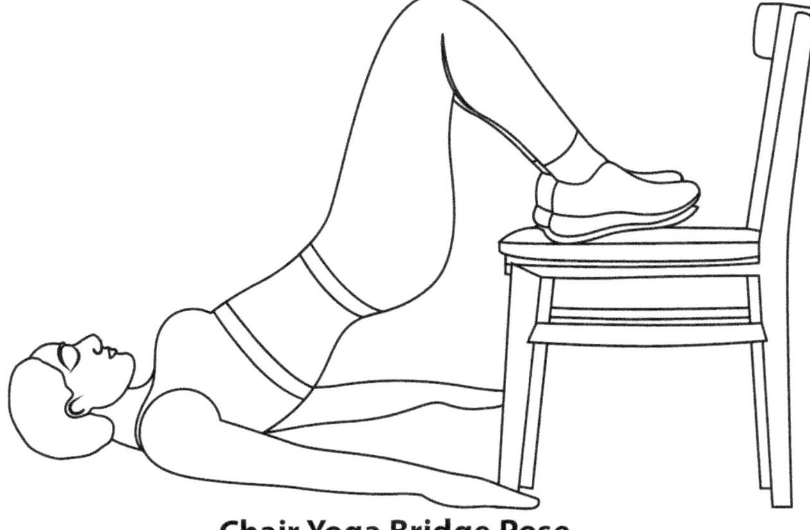

Chair Yoga Bridge Pose

1. Sit on the floor in front of a chair with your knees bent.
2. Lie down on your back, making sure your head is directly in line with the chair.
3. Bend your elbows slightly and place your palms flat on the floor beside your hips, fingertips pointing towards your feet.
4. Lift your legs and place your feet on the chair with knees bent. Adjust your body as required to get the positioning.
5. Inhale, push down flat on the chair with your feet and against the floor with your shoulders to lift up your hips.
6. Engage your midsection, pull your belly in, exhale as you lift your hips up as high as it's comfortable for you.
7. Take slow, deep breaths, allowing your chest to expand with each inhale and releasing any tension with each exhale.

8. Hold the pose for about 4-6 breaths, feeling the stretch across your chest, hips and thighs.
9. To come out of the pose, exhale as you slowly lower your hips back down to the mat.
10. Rest seated in a comfortable position, allowing your body to integrate the benefits of the pose.

CHAPTER 7: CHAIR YOGA RELAXATION AND COOL DOWN EXERCISES

Finding serenity after a session of chair yoga practice is just as important as the movement itself. This chapter guides you through gentle relaxation and cool-down exercises to help your body and mind fully unwind.

Preparing For Relaxation

1. **Find a Quiet Space:** Choose a comfortable spot in your home where you can relax undisturbed. Ideally, this space will be free from clutter and have a calming atmosphere.
2. **Adjust Your Chair:** Sit comfortably in your chair with feet placed flat on the floor, at about hip-width apart. Ensure your back is supported, and you can easily lengthen your spine. You can use a rolled towel or small pillow for added support in your lower back if needed.
3. **Soften Your Gaze:** Close your eyes gently, or if you prefer, soften your gaze by focusing on a single point in the room. Take a couple of deep breaths, inhaling slowly through the nose and exhaling completely through your mouth.

Gentle Stretches For Cooling Down

1. **Neck Rolls:** Begin by gently rolling your head in a circular motion, five times forward and five times backward. Feel the tension release in your neck muscles.
2. **Shoulder Rolls:** Roll your shoulders forward in small circles five times, followed by five backward circles.

3. **Seated Arm Circles:** Stretch out your arms at shoulder height to the sides. Make small forward circles for ten breaths, then reverse direction and make small backward circles for ten breaths.
4. **Seated Ankle Circles:** Point your toes and rotate your ankles clockwise for ten circles, then counter-clockwise for ten circles. Repeat on the other foot.
5. **Seated Forward Fold:** Slowly hinge at the hips and fold forward, reaching your hands towards the floor or your shins. Breathe deeply and hold for several breaths, allowing your back to round naturally. If you feel any discomfort, simply adjust the position or come up slightly.
6. **Seated Side Bends:** Inhale and reach your right arm overhead. As you exhale, gently side bend your torso to the left, reaching your left hand towards the floor or the side of your chair. Hold for several breaths and repeat the bend on the other side.

Restorative Poses For Deep Relaxation

1. **Supported Child's Pose:** Sit on a chair with a folded blanket or pillow placed on your laps. Lean forward, resting your, head, torso and arms comfortably on the blanket or pillow. Alternatively, allow your hands to drape towards the floor. Breathe deeply and hold for several minutes.
2. **Supported Legs-Up-the-Wall Pose:** Lie on the floor on your back with your legs extended straight up the wall. If the full pose feels uncomfortable, you can bend your knees slightly. Place a rolled towel or blanket under your lower back for added support. Breathe deeply and hold for several minutes.

1. **Body Scan:** Close your eyes and focus your attention on each part of your body, starting with your toes and gradually moving upwards. Notice any areas of tension and consciously relax those muscles. Breathe deeply and visualize a wave of relaxation washing over you.
2. **Visualization:** Imagine yourself in a peaceful and calming environment, such as a beach or a serene forest. Engage your senses by picturing the sights, sounds, and smells of this place. Allow yourself to feel completely relaxed and at peace.
3. **Deep Breathing Exercises:** Practice slow, deep breathing throughout your relaxation period. Inhale through your nose while counting to four, then hold for a count of two, and slowly exhale through the mouth for a count of six. Repeat this breathing pattern for several minutes.

Ending Your Practice

When you're ready to come out of your relaxation, breathe deeply a few times and gently wiggle your toes and fingers. Slowly roll your head from side to side and open your eyes at your own pace. Take a moment to appreciate the sense of calm and well-being that your chair yoga practice has brought you.

Additional Tips

- **Set a Timer:** If you tend to lose track of time during relaxation, set a gentle timer to remind you when your practice is complete.
- **Focus on Gratitude:** Take a moment to express gratitude for your body and its ability to move and find stillness.
- **Incorporate Music:** Play calming music during your relaxation period to create a peaceful atmosphere.

- **Make it a Habit:** Aim to make chair yoga relaxation and cool-down exercises part of your daily routine for optimal benefits.

By taking the time to unwind after your chair yoga practice, you can deepen the mind-body connection, improve sleep quality, and manage stress more effectively. Remember, chair yoga is a journey of self-discovery and exploration. Listen to your body, find what feels good for you, and enjoy the process of nurturing your well-being.

CHAPTER 8: CHAIR YOGA AND MEDITATION: CULTIVATING INNER PEACE

Chair yoga, with its focus on gentle movement and breath awareness, is a natural gateway to meditation. This chapter explores the benefits of meditation and how it can be seamlessly integrated into your chair yoga practice.

Meditation is an ancient practice that cultivates a state of focused attention and inner calm. By quieting the mind and observing your thoughts and emotions without judgment, you can experience a sense of peace and well-being that extends beyond the yoga mat, impacting your daily life.

Benefits Of Meditation

- **Reduced Stress and Anxiety:** Meditation helps calm the body's stress response system, lowering cortisol levels and promoting a sense of relaxation.
- **Improved Focus and Concentration:** Regular meditation practice can enhance your ability to reduce distractions and be more focused on the present moment.
- **Enhanced Self-Awareness:** Through meditation, you develop an understanding of your thoughts, physical sensations and emotions at a deeper level.
- **Improved Sleep Quality:** Meditation can promote better sleep by calming the mind and reducing racing thoughts before bed.
- **Increased Emotional Regulation:** Meditation equips you with tools for managing difficult emotions and responding to challenges with greater clarity.

Mindfulness And Chair Yoga

Chair yoga, by its very nature, fosters mindfulness — the practice of a judgment free awareness of the present moment. As you move your body with awareness and focus on your breathing, you naturally cultivate a state of quiet focus. This mindful state transitions beautifully into seated meditation.

Basic Meditation Poses for Beginners

- **Seated Mountain Pose (Tadasana):** Sit tall in your chair with feet placed flat on the floor, at about hip-width apart. Lengthen your spine and keep your shoulders relaxed. Rest your hands gently on your lap or thighs with palms facing down.
- **Supported Child's Pose (Balasana with Chair):** Sit on a chair with a pillow or folded blanket placed on your laps. Lean forward, resting your, head, torso and arms comfortably on the blanket or pillow. Alternatively, allow your hands to drape towards the floor. Breathe deeply and hold for several minutes.

Advanced Meditation Techniques

- **Body Scan Meditation:** Sit comfortably then focus your attention one by one on parts of the body, beginning with your toes and gradually moving upwards. Notice any sensations without judgment and mentally let go of any tension you find.
- **Guided Visualization:** Engage your senses by picturing yourself in a peaceful and calming environment. Imagine the sights, sounds, and smells of this place, allowing yourself to feel completely relaxed and at peace.

- **Mantra Meditation:** Choose a simple mantra (a word or phrase) and silently repeat it to yourself with each breath. This helps focus the mind and quiet background thoughts.

Meditation And Your Daily Routine

Just like chair yoga, incorporating meditation into your routine daily can significantly impact your overall well-being. Here's how to make it a habit:

- **Start Small:** Begin with just a few minutes of meditation daily and increase the duration gradually as it becomes more comfortable.
- **Find a Quiet Space:** Select a quiet and clutter-free space in your home where you won't be interrupted.
- **Set a Timer:** Use a timer to avoid checking the clock and remain focused on your practice.
- **Be Kind to Yourself:** Don't get discouraged if your find your mind wandering during meditation. Simply acknowledge the wandering thought and gently bring back your attention to the present moment.
- **Meditate with Others:** Consider joining a meditation group or finding a meditation app with guided practices to enhance your experience.

Remember, meditation is a journey, not a destination. Embrace the practice with patience and kindness towards yourself. As you integrate meditation into your chair yoga routine, you'll discover a deeper sense of calm and inner peace that will nourish your mind, body, and spirit.

CHAPTER 9: NUTRITION AND LIFESTYLE: FUELING YOUR CHAIR YOGA JOURNEY

Your chair yoga practice is a wonderful way to enhance your physical and mental well-being. But just like fuel is needed by a car for smooth running, your body also thrives with proper nourishment and healthy lifestyle choices. This chapter explores key areas that, when combined with your chair yoga routine, can optimize your overall health and vitality.

Staying Hydrated: The Foundation of Health

Water is the single most important nutrient for your body. It plays a crucial role in every bodily function, from regulating temperature to lubricating joints and transporting nutrients. Here's how staying hydrated can support your chair yoga practice:

- **Improved Flexibility:** Dehydration can stiffen muscles and limit your range of motion. Drinking enough water keeps your muscles supple and helps you move with greater ease during your chair yoga poses.
- **Enhanced Energy Levels:** Feeling sluggish during your practice? Dehydration can zap your energy. Proper hydration ensures your body functions efficiently, allowing you to participate in your chair yoga routine with more vigor.
- **Reduced Risk of Dizziness:** Dehydration can cause dizziness and lightheadedness, especially during movements that involve changes in position. Staying hydrated helps you stay focused and prevents these potential safety concerns.

Tips for Staying Hydrated:

- **Carry a reusable water bottle:** Keep a water bottle at hand throughout the day and aim to take frequent sips.
- **Flavor it Up:** Add slices of lemon, cucumber, or berries to your water for a refreshing twist.
- **Choose water-rich foods:** Fruits and vegetables like watermelon, cantaloupe, spinach, and celery are naturally high in water content and contribute to your daily hydration needs.
- **Monitor your urine color:** Pale yellow urine indicates good hydration. Darker urine suggests you might need to drink more fluids.
- **Listen to your body:** Don't wait until you feel thirsty to drink. Aim to consistently drink water all through the day, even if you don't feel parched.

Sleep And Relaxation: Recharging Your Batteries

Adequate sleep is essential for both physical and mental recovery. It allows your body to repair tissues, strengthen your immune system, and consolidate memories. Here's how getting enough sleep benefits your chair yoga practice:

- **Improved Muscle Repair:** Deep sleep is crucial for muscle growth and repair. Proper rest ensures your muscles recover effectively from your chair yoga exercises, allowing you to feel stronger and more energized for your next session.
- **Enhanced Cognitive Function:** Sleep deprivation can impair your focus and balance. A good night's sleep sharpens your mind and improves your coordination, both of which are beneficial for your chair yoga practice.
- **Reduced Stress and Anxiety:** Chronic stress can lead to muscle tension and hinder your ability to relax during your practice. Getting enough sleep helps you manage stress more effectively and promotes a sense of calm, allowing you to fully benefit from the relaxation aspect of chair yoga.

Tips for a Good Night's Sleep:

- **Establish a regular sleep schedule:** Go to bed and wake up at consistent times, even on weekends. This helps regulate your body's natural sleep-wake cycle.
- **Create a relaxing bedtime routine:** Engage in calming activities before bed, such as taking a warm bath, reading a book, or practicing gentle stretches. Avoid watching television or using electronic devices for at least an hour before sleep.
- **Optimize your sleep environment:** Ensure your bedroom is dark, quiet, and cool. Invest in a comfortable mattress and pillows to promote restful sleep.
- **Limit caffeine and alcohol intake:** While a morning cup of coffee might be a part of your routine, avoid excessive caffeine intake, especially in the afternoon and evening. Similarly, limit alcohol consumption as it can cause a disruption of your sleep cycle.
- **Regular exercise:** Regular physical activity, like your chair yoga practice, can improve sleep quality. However, avoid strenuous exercise close to bedtime.

Diet And Eating Right: Nourishing Your Body

The food you choose plays a vital role in your overall health and well-being. Eating a balanced diet provides the body with the essential nutrients it needs to function optimally and supports your chair yoga practice in the following ways:

- **Increased Energy Levels:** A balanced diet rich in whole grains, fruits, vegetables, and lean protein ensures a steady supply of energy throughout the day. This can help you to feel more energized during your chair yoga practice.
- **Improved Strength and Stamina:** Eating enough protein helps build and maintain muscle mass. Consuming a variety

of healthy fats also provides your body with sustained energy for your chair yoga routine.

- **Weight Management:** Maintaining a healthy weight can reduce stress on your joints and improve your overall balance and flexibility, making it easier to perform chair yoga poses.

Tips for a Healthy Diet:

- **Focus on whole foods:** Prioritize whole grains, fruits, vegetables, lean protein sources (like fish, chicken, or beans), and healthy fats (such as avocado, seeds and nuts) in your diet. These foods are packed with essential nutrients that are needed for your body to thrive.

- **Limit processed foods:** Processed foods are often high in unhealthy fats, added sugars, and sodium. These can contribute to weight gain and other health problems. Opt for fresh, whole foods whenever possible.
- **Plan your meals:** Planning your meals and snacks in advance can help you make healthy choices and avoid unhealthy temptations.
- **Read food labels:** Pay attention to serving sizes and the nutrient content listed on food labels. This can help you make informed choices about what you eat.
- **Portion control:** Practice mindful eating and pay attention to your hunger cues. Avoid overeating and aim for moderate portions to maintain a healthy weight.
- **Stay Hydrated:** As mentioned earlier, staying hydrated is crucial for good health and digestion. Drinking plenty of water helps you feel full and can prevent overeating.
- **Don't deprive yourself:** Allow yourself occasional treats in moderation. A balanced approach to eating is key to long-term success.

By incorporating these nutritional tips into your lifestyle, you can nourish your body from the inside out and optimize your chair yoga practice for greater well-being. Remember, a healthy diet is not about deprivation; it's about making conscious choices that fuel your body and support your overall health.

- **Talk to your physician:** If you have any underlying health conditions or take medications, consult your doctor before making any significant changes to your diet or exercise routine. They can guide you on a personalized approach to healthy living.
- **Listen to your body:** Start paying attention to how your body reacts to certain foods. If you sense any digestive discomfort or feel sluggish after eating, adjust your diet accordingly.
- **Make Gradual Changes:** Don't try to overhaul your diet overnight. Introduce healthy changes gradually and focus on making them sustainable for the long term.

Remember, a healthy lifestyle combined with your chair yoga practice is a powerful recipe for optimal well-being. By nourishing your body and mind, you can embrace a life filled with vitality and joy as you move through your golden years.

CHAPTER 10: CHALLENGE YOURSELF: 28-DAY CHAIR YOGA JOURNEY FOR SENIORS

This 28-day chair yoga challenge is designed to gently guide you through a progressive sequence of poses, starting with beginner-friendly movements and gradually increasing the intensity as you build more strength and confidence. Each day offers a short practice (around 10-15 minutes) that you can comfortably incorporate into your daily routine.

Important Note: Listen to your body throughout this challenge. If you feel any pain or discomfort, adjust the poses or take a rest day. It's important to progress at your own pace and prioritize safety above all else.

Week 1: Building a Foundation (Beginner Poses)

- **Day 1:** Seated Cat-Cow Pose (Marjaryasana-Bitilasana) & Chair Mountain Pose (Tadasana) - Focus on gentle spine mobility and proper posture.
- **Day 2:** Seated Arm Circles & Seated Shoulder Rolls - Improve upper body mobility and range of motion.
- **Day 3:** Seated Warrior II Pose (Virabhadrasana II) - Strengthen legs and core while exploring basic balance techniques.
- **Day 4:** Seated Side Stretches - Enhance flexibility in the side body and core.
- **Day 5:** Seated Forward Fold (Paschimottanasana) - Improve hamstring flexibility and promote relaxation.
- **Day 6:** Rest & Review - Reflect on the past week's practice and how your body feels.

Week 2: Exploring Stability (Beginner to Intermediate Poses)

- **Day 7:** Chair Supported Tree Pose (Vrksasana) - Challenge your balance with this supported single-leg pose.
- **Day 8:** Seated Twists (Parivrtta Tadasana) - Introduce gentle twisting motions to increase spinal mobility.
- **Day 9:** Chair Revolved Side Stretch With Arm Reach - Open your chest and core while exploring a gentle twist with chair support.
- **Day 10:** Seated Eagle Pose (Garudasana) (Modification) - Improve balance and coordination with a modified version of Eagle Pose.
- **Day 11:** Chair Supported Downward-Facing Dog (Adho Mukha Svanasana) (Modification) - Gently stretch your hamstrings and spine with chair support.
- **Day 12:** Rest & Review - Celebrate your progress and acknowledge any areas of improvement.

Week 3: Reaching New Heights (Intermediate Poses)

- **Day 13:** Standing Side Bends with Chair Support - Increase side body flexibility with chair support.
- **Day 14:** Chair Supported Warrior III Pose (Virabhadrasana III) (Modification) - Challenge your balance and strengthen your core with extended leg variations.
- **Day 15:** Seated Pigeon Pose (Eka Pada Rajakapotasana) (Modification) - Improve hip flexibility with a supported variation of Pigeon Pose.
- **Day 16:** Chair Half Moon Pose
- **Day 17:** Chair Sun Salutation Sequence
- **Day 18:** Rest & Review - Re-evaluate your progress and celebrate your achievements.

- **Day 19:** Chair Revolved Side Stretch With Arm Reach
- **Day 20:** Standing Warrior III Pose (Virabhadrasana III) - Challenge your balance with a full standing Warrior III pose.
- **Day 21:** Chair Pigeon Pose (Eka Pada Rajakapotasana) - Practice a deeper version of Pigeon Pose with chair support.
- **Day 22:** Half Moon Pose (Ardha Chandrasana) (Modification) - Explore this balancing pose with chair support (optional).
- **Day 23:** Chair Supported Bridge Pose
- **Day 24:** Rest & Review - Take a moment to appreciate your journey and newfound skills.

- **Day 25:** Review & Repeat - Choose your favorite poses from the challenge and create a personalized practice routine.
- **Day 26:** Explore New Poses - Use online resources or a chair yoga class to learn new poses at your own pace, focusing on maintaining your newfound strength and flexibility.

- **Day 27:** Rest & Reflect - Take a well-deserved rest day and reflect on the positive changes you've experienced through this challenge.
- **Day 28:** Celebrate & Commit - Celebrate your accomplishment and commit to incorporating chair yoga into your ongoing wellness routine!

Congratulations! You've successfully completed the 28-day chair yoga challenge. Remember, consistency is key. By continuing to regularly practice chair yoga, you can maintain the benefits you've gained and keep exploring new ways to move your body with grace and ease.

Bonus Tips:

- **Find a Chair Yoga Community:** Consider joining a chair yoga class or online community to connect with others on a similar journey, share experiences, and stay motivated.

- **Track Your Progress:** Keeping a simple journal to track your progress can be a great way to stay motivated and celebrate your achievements.
- **Listen to Your Body:** Always prioritize safety and adjust poses as needed. Don't hesitate to take rest days or modify poses when your body needs it.
- **Most Importantly, Have Fun!** Chair yoga is a joyful practice that allows you to move your body, connect with your breath, and experience the joy of movement at any age.

END